Vibrant Child

7 Steps to Increase Your Child's Health & Happiness

Mike & Amanda Hinman

Vibrant Child

Printed by:
Hinman Holistic Health Institute, Ltd.
2013 Chinkapin Oak Dr.
Mt. Prospect, IL 60056
www.hinmans.com

Published in the United States of America

Book ID: 160219-00351

ISBN-13: 978-0-9975380-0-7

Praise for Vibrant Child

I am insanely impressed that this book is filled with such high quality and helpful content. I will not only be reading it again and again to try to work through these steps in our lives, but I would recommend this as a resource to every family I know. I think it is phenomenal. Courtney Digate - Chicago

Vibrant Child is a lot more than a book. It is a mission of two parents who, having gone through their own year of hell, came out inspired to help other families. I highly recommend this book for its heart just as much as its content. Allen Vaysberg, Life Recalibration Expert and author of *The New Love Triangle - Your practical guide to a love-filled life!*

A must read for ALL parents. Mike and Amanda dedicate their lives and business to helping parents support their children through difficulties, illness, and symptoms. I truly believe their message, and Vibrant Child: 7 Steps to Increase Your Childs Health and Happiness, should be on every parent's nightstand. This book talks about the root causes for the toughest challenges facing parents today like ADHD, Diabetes, and Auto-immune conditions. By the end you will not only understand what problems are occurring but why. Taking it a step further the Hinman Holistic Health Institute and their various programs show you how to support any family through every challenge. Revolutionizing parenting to focus on a whole health, whole family, and whole life model that we all so deeply desire. Jessica Shada - Colorado

I think it's great you wrote this book for parents that are looking for education on how to help their children live a happier more vibrant life. I think it'll be very helpful to many people. It is an easy read, like listening in on an interesting conversation. Jennifer Chan, MD - Midwest Center for Women's Healthcare

Contents

Dedication

We dedicate this book to our parents who have supported our girls and us in all stages of our lives, even when things were rough or they didn't understand our perspectives. Also, to all parents that are doing their best every day to care for our most precious asset, our children…our future.

Introduction

This book builds the argument that it is possible for children to improve their health and happiness in any situation. You'll discover how the three most common things parents worry about (picky eating, hyper-sensitivity and difficulty concentrating) are related and can all be reversed. In addition, this book demonstrates there is support for families experiencing more significant health challenges, like the ones we faced, and gives you a reason to be optimistic. Transformation begins when parents understand the dramatic changes that have affected three aspects of life today:

1. **How we eat** – Food is information for our bodies. Because our bodies are constantly regenerating, the information we give our bodies via food affects the way they function. The food supply in the United States has changed more in the past 20 years than it had in the prior 200 years. Therefore, most Americans are literally eating different foods today, and our bodies don't know how to process this information. By focusing on eating real foods, in their natural state, a person can dramatically improve his health.

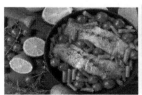

Photo from Understanding Food Labels

2. **How we live** – The world around us is full of information. Everything in our environment is perceived through senses, which trigger responses in the brain. Therefore, it is essential to understand how our environment impacts our health. Did you know that the average person today takes in more stimuli through their senses in one 24-hour period than our parents did in a year when they were young? That means our children are literally taking in more information in one year than our great-grandparents did in their entire lives. All of these stimuli affect our body, so it is imperative to know how to balance it in order to achieve optimal health and happiness.

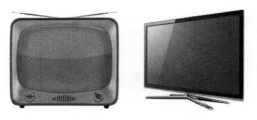

3. **How we learn** – Children today spend an average of over 500 additional hours each year in structured activities than in the 1980s. This includes changes in the public academic environment as well as activities such as sports, music lessons and homework. As a result there is less time for unstructured creativity in our children's lives. We will share how the lack of creativity can lead to chronic negative stress, which is very detrimental to health.

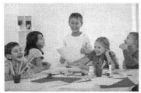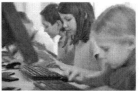

The combination of changes in these three areas leaves a potential for our lives to become unbalanced. Imbalances cause either physical or emotional challenges, which ultimately leave a person unhealthy and unhappy. However, by understanding what has changed and how to collaborate with our world in the 21st century, we can live a truly vibrant life and guide our children to do it too.

It is important to note that the information in this book is not intended to discredit or demean the work of other professionals, such as medical doctors, therapists, educators, or other specialists. These people work very hard to help the people they serve. This information is meant to act as a complement to any other service, because it provides a holistic approach to health and happiness.

Mike & Amanda

Chapter 1

Support for Parents

Mike and Amanda Hinman are the founders of Hinman Holistic Health Institute, Ltd. They work with parents who seek to maximize the health and happiness of their families. They live in the Chicagoland area with their four young daughters. This book is a way to share their message and is written interview style with Kelly, mother of two, living in Chicago.

Kelly: Why did you write Vibrant Child: 7 Steps to Increase Your Child's Health and Happiness?

Mike: We wrote the book because we had our own year from hell and came out the other side stronger than ever. We understand that parents want what's best for their children. Some parents will pick up this book because they want to learn more about how to support their child's best health and happiness. These parents may have a nagging concern, or occasional random thoughts, such as:

- My kids are picky eaters and don't seem interested in eating well; how do I get them to care?

- My child is hyper-sensitive about things; why does she react so strongly?

- My son is forgetful; how can I help him focus better?

- Can allergies and gut health affect my child's emotional health too?

- My child seems unsure of himself; how can I help boost his self-esteem?

- My kids seem happy, but how can I gauge their overall health?

- Experts don't agree on health topics; how do I know what to focus on as a parent?

- What are early warning signs of anxiety in kids?

- How much do food and diet relate to behavior and sensory issues?

- I worry about how our family history of heart disease, cholesterol, depression, alcoholism, and so on, will affect my children. How can I support my children to prevent these conditions?

- What can I learn to support my daughter's health and body image as she gets older and stress increases?

Other parents may pick up this book because there is a specific, impactful situation affecting their child that they wish was different. First of all, I want you to know that everything is going to be all right. You are in a good spot, being the best parent you can be, and if you are in a tough place right now, we are going to help you get through this.

Throughout this book, we share knowledge, inspiration, and practical strategies that will empower any parent, whether currently facing a difficult situation with a child or proactively seeking out a comprehensive, yet simple way to approach guiding a family to live its best life.

Our family has been in a really tough place and bounced back with more health and happiness than we even thought possible. The good news is we have spent a lot of money and years of our lives sifting through the boatloads of conflicting information to bring you a straightforward approach to guiding your child. It dramatically helped our family, and I am positive it will do the same for yours. In fact, it is our belief that almost all personal health and happiness challenges can be eliminated by taking a closer look at how we **eat**, how we **live**, and how we **learn**.

Kelly: It seems like we are going to talk about a lot of information, but you make it sound manageable, which is reassuring. I have a six-year-old daughter named Kate, and sometimes I worry, because she seems very sensitive. She reacts to the littlest things and gets very upset, so when you mentioned the connection between gut health and emotional health, this is something that has crossed my mind. Also, my eight-year-old son Dylan is very active, and loves his friends. He doesn't mind going to school because of the social aspect, but I wonder if he's able to stay focused and get the most out of his learning. I'm happy to hear that I will learn some helpful information to support my kids. It appears that this book will also be helpful to parents who have more difficult situations, as well.

Amanda: Yes, in fact, we work with parents who have concerns because their children struggle with ADD, ADHD, anxiety, autism, allergies, an auto-immune condition, diabetes, digestive distress, sensory defensiveness, seizures, or other situations that make them feel different.

You may want to take a deep breath for this first bit because it can get a little heavy. Hopefully, you are in a situation where you can only partially relate to these feelings. If so, that means you are much farther ahead of where we started off. Rest assured that if you do feel all of the things we describe, and more, you're in the right place, because we've been in your shoes.

Mike: We know how stress over a situation with one child can affect your marriage, your other kids, your work…basically, it affects your whole life.

Amanda: It's true. Perhaps you lose sleep because you are worried about your child. You wonder if you are doing everything you can to provide the best life possible for him. The memories that stand out are when you watch your son break into uncontrollable giggles because he thought the dog was funny, or when you see your daughter's face light as she learned to ride her bike for the first time. It's those moments of pure joy that tug at your heart. But lately, you have been noticing them less and less. Your child seems to be upset more often, quick to anger…overall, less confident in himself. He may be struggling with either a physical or emotional situation that is making life tough.

You are doing your best to show your child he is loved for who he is. You are the mom who drives to and from soccer practices, you help study for the spelling tests, read books before bed, and watch dance recitals and swim meets with a recorder in hand. You feel your heart break when you discover that your child has a circumstance that is making his life tough. You are afraid for what this means, and feel sad thinking about the missed opportunities and future limitations. You want what is best for your child, and somewhere deep in your heart you know there must be another way to empower your child, even when the experts say this is the best you can do. You have been told you are doing everything you can and that your child will learn to live with his condition. But something doesn't settle with you. To make things worse, you may feel totally frustrated with your husband, because he just doesn't seem to understand that this current situation is not going to work. You're tired of the fact that he doesn't see that there has to be something else going on, something more you can do.

Does this sound familiar? Ever think… "No one gets what I *know* about my child"?

Most moms do. So we start doubting what's in our hearts. When we tune out our intuition, we feel lost and scared. And when we feel lost and scared, we STRESS OUT!

Kelly: Wow, my heart goes out to anyone feeling what you describe. I haven't been faced with a situation quite like that, but can definitely relate to some of it. Especially the part about my husband being on a different page. Mike, what's a dad's perspective?

Mike: Now, Dads are a little different. Many fathers out there believe stress is a made-up word your doctor uses when he has no idea what is wrong with you. They believe the word "holistic" is only associated with vegetarian hippies who think all the world's problems could be solved with love. Some

Dads are counting down the minutes until their next round of golf with the guys, imagining the first puff of a stogie, the sound a beer makes when you first open the can, and thinking about how good it's going to taste. Regardless of what your wife thinks you know, this beer is your salvation and the perfect way of dealing with stress. She just doesn't get it. Guys are different, and have a much simpler approach to life.

When you hear from the teacher that your child skips problems on the math worksheet or can't sit still at his desk, you think they are just being a kid, it's a boy being a boy, and you did the same things growing up and turned out just fine.

When your daughter freaks out about what clothes to put on in the morning, you think she's just being pain in the ass and you don't understand girls. Your only thought is maybe I need to put my foot down more at home, because these kids are spoiled.

Then it escalates to the point where you learn from a professional that your child has a condition, such as ADHD, sensory defensiveness, or whatever situation is affecting them. You think, okay, what does this mean, what's the next step? If the doctor recommends taking medication or going to occupational therapy, then that's what we do.

But what happens when, even with the medicine or therapy, your child has less laughter and more sadness? He is constantly feeling different from his friends, and it's affecting his self-esteem? What happens when your child refuses to eat anything that is even remotely healthy, and as much as you hate to admit it, you don't like to think about how that might affect their health in 30 years. You are willing to do whatever it takes to be the best Dad you can and build up your child. You just need an answer that is proven to work, not the unconventional philosophies that your wife talks about.

Amanda: Consider this – what if Mom started to listen to her heart? What if you followed your heart and found a place to learn what is happening inside your child's body? What if you believed it's possible to heal using real foods, to balance your emotions, to feel confident instead of worried, and to laugh every day? Now, what if your child believed it, too?

Mike: Consider this – what if Dad could step into the lead and know with certainty that there is something different he could to do help his child? What if he saw proof and trusted in an approach that had no negative side effects, only upside potential? It's a sure bet.

What if your child….

- Walked into a room with her head held high?

- Was able to brush off a teammate's rude outburst?

- Looked in the mirror and loved what she saw?

- Didn't have fears about missing the ball when at bat?

- Talked excitedly about what he learned in school?

- Didn't worry about getting a low score on a math test?

- Was able to wait calmly while his younger sister tried to spell cat?

- Laughed even more?

- Slept through the night?

Amanda: Suddenly your life is really happy! You no longer feel stressed out and worried about your child and you notice that your whole family is happier too. Your family life is now fun, connected, and exciting!

Kelly: That sounds great. I definitely want those things for my children and family.

Chapter 2

Why This Book Is Different

Kelly: I feel like there are so many resources available now to help children. There are so many different specialists – from doctors like pediatric endocrinologists, pediatric neurologists, and neurofeedback specialists, to other experts like psychotherapists, occupational therapists, chiropractors, school counselors, etc. You name it, and there is someone who can help a child. What's different about this book?

Amanda: You are absolutely right about the number of services and people that are available to help our children. In fact, many of these services and people are incredibly valuable resources, but it can be overwhelming. Each person you go to will tell you what action you should take to help your child.

It's easy to become busy focusing on what to do to support your child – take them to appointments with doctors and specialists, participate in weekly therapy or tutoring sessions, create a specific Individualized Education Program (IEP) at school, etc. Although many of these things are helpful, and do provide great benefit to our kids, oftentimes parents feel like they are just taking the advice of experts without really understanding *why* the situation came about in the first place.

Our intention with this book is to help parents uncover the reason *why*. This is the deeper reason for their child's struggling. Whether it is a challenge for your child to eat healthily, or a challenge for your child to handle an unpredictable situation, there is always a cause for the behavior. Once parents know on a deep level *why* things are the way they are, they can decide more clearly *what* action is the best for their child and their family. The last piece, implementing *how* to change, is dramatically easier when everyone is certain why and what to do first. In other words, reading this book and learning why will make it easier to move forward in working with doctors, therapists, schools, coaches, and others, because parents have amazing clarity.

Mike: Understanding why things are happening puts you in a place of empowerment and allows you to take the lead in your child's healthcare and education. It's amazing how much things change when you're sitting in a doctors' office or at your child's school conference, and you have a deep understanding of why things are happening. All of a sudden you can objectively evaluate and decide what will work and what won't. How many times have you met with someone who is providing recommendations about your child's well-being, and received their recommendations, but didn't really understand how the recommendations were supposed to help?

Sometimes we do things just because the person in the white coat said that's what we need to do. Now, I'm not suggesting you don't need to listen to your doctor, therapist, or teacher, but what if you could be an equal participant in the decision-making process, because you understood why things were happening and what was affecting your child? What if you could listen with appreciation to their suggestions and feel confident about deciding whether their recommendations would be valuable to you or not?

Not too long ago, I was shopping for a new backpack. There were certain features I was looking for but I was having such a difficult time finding one bag that had everything I wanted. Because of this problem, it took some time to find what I wanted. In fact, it should never take anyone this long to buy a backpack, ever. Night after night, Amanda would constantly poke fun at me for Googling backpacks yet again. I knew why I wanted the backpack and all of the things I wanted it to include. Instead of taking someone else's recommendation, I did my homework. It bordered on insanity, but the point here is that because of all my homework, I ended up buying exactly what I wanted, and I was 100% confident in the purchase. Now imagine having that feeling when it comes to something important, like the health of your child.

Kelly: I'm with you, feeling empowered is definitely what I want. I have to be honest, I didn't want to think about questioning things our pediatrician or teachers recommend. That seems overwhelming. Are you suggesting that I should do that more often?

Amanda: I think each person has to answer that question for herself. By no means is the intention to make your life overwhelming by feeling skeptical about everything around you. However, no one wants an outfielder like this when a big hitter is up to bat:

11

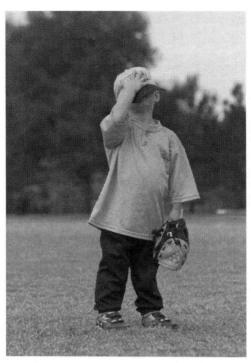

What is so frustrating for parents, at least it was for me, is that when life throws you a curve ball and someone's health is impacted, many times it feels like it came out of left field. The reality is that there are numerous ways our bodies give signals well before a major imbalance comes up. **When parents approach raising children from a place of curiosity, and stop to ask themselves what the best fit is for their child, the child feels understood.** As parents, you know the MOST about your children and always will. Each child is unique, and requires a personalized approach to living his healthiest and happiest life.

Kelly: That really makes sense. When I am able to understand why Kate is so sensitive and why Dylan is more interested in his sports than learning at school, it will be easier to make empowered decisions and work together with their teachers, coaches, doctors, and therapists. I understand how unique each child is. My kids are completely different, and you're making me think how they may benefit from different health recommendations, just like teachers differentiate in some of the learning experiences in school. So how do I learn why my kids behave the way they do?

Amanda: We like to think of this as uncovering the *Level 3 Why*. It's funny, because the Level 3 Why is something three and four-year-old kids do naturally. Like the time when my inquisitive niece Kaitlin asked her mom, "Why do the clouds move?" Her mom responded, "Because the wind blows them." Then Kaitlin asked, "Why does the wind blow them?" The next response was "Because it's strong and that's how our weather changes." Then came the question, "Why does the weather change?" You get the point. How many times can you remember saying "Because I said so!"? It's like we have been programmed from a young age to stop asking why and just trust someone else. However, the key to our personal health and happiness comes when we uncover why for ourselves, and allow our kids to do it, too. Just like an iceberg, from the surface you only know what you feel, but by looking a little deeper, you discover the underlying cause and the *Level 3 Why*.

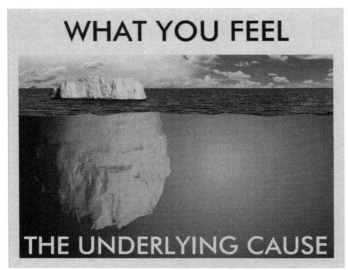

Image courtesy of truehealthct.com

Here's an example of the Level 3 Why for a child who is struggling with Attention Deficit Disorder (ADD). The first question, why is he diagnosed with ADD, is because he has a variety of symptoms, including difficulty staying focused. The second level, why is he not able to stay focused, could be related to unbalanced serotonin and dopamine levels in his brain. This is where most doctors, psychotherapists, and other specialists are really helpful. Typically, either through diagnostic testing, observation or other formative assessment they can identify the underlying reason for a situation. However, the Level 3 Why is why are his serotonin and dopamine levels unbalanced? In many cases, the answer is originally because of genetics.

Here is where the true potential comes in! The field of epigenetics now proves that our health outcomes are a result of lifestyle factors, rather than heredity.

The definition of epigenetics is the study of the process by which genetic information is translated into the substance and behavior of an organism. In other words, just because a person inherited a predisposition for a certain circumstance, such as anxiety, ADD, ADHD, autism, auto-immune disease, allergies, cancer, diabetes, heart disease, and so on, whether or not that condition is activated depends on the person's lifestyle choices. Almost all modern conditions are *epigenetic,* not genetic. Dr. Kelly Brogan, a practicing psychiatrist and author of *A Mind of Your Own*, describes it like this:

"Even though genes encoded by DNA are more or less static (barring the occurrence of mutation), the expression of those genes can be highly dynamic in response to environmental influences. Epigenetics, defined more technically, is the study of sections of your DNA (called "marks", or "markers") that essentially tell your genes when and how strongly to express themselves. Like conductors of an orchestra, these epigenetic marks control not only your health and longevity, but also how you pass your genes on to future generations."[1]

By helping our children uncover the Level 3 Why of an imbalance they experience in their lives, then guiding them to make lifestyle changes, we are creating not only healthier and happier lives for our children, but also for our grandchildren. This is great news for any parents who are worried about a family legacy of illness or health challenges. When you take a closer look at the way your children eat, the way they live, and the way they learn, you will know how to guide them to a different destiny. Dr. Mercola, an osteopathic physician who is board-certified in family medicine, says, "Now we realize our fate is not sealed at the twining of our double helix, we avail ourselves of a whole new world of possibilities. There are things we can do to *change our genetics,* and therefore our health."[2]

An analogy that is helpful to think of the impact of epigenetics is to think of a dozen eggs. When you are born, your genetic DNA is like a carton of raw eggs. There is structure, and certain elements of the eggs will always be present, but the potential for what those eggs can become is unlimited. You can turn those eggs into an omelet, a carbonara pasta dinner, a cake, or meatloaf. The point is that you are not stuck with raw eggs to eat simply because that is what you started with.

Kelly: So you're telling me that my children's health and happiness depends on how they eat, how they live, and how they learn? It's not because that's the way they were born; it's how they've always been?

Mike: You got it! In this book, we provide parents the chance to consider new perspectives on things like food, love, sleep, activity, creativity, and spirituality, which are all part of your child's daily life. This is the part where some people feel a little edgy; I used to, as well. No one wants to be told that they have to eat better, sleep more, and stress less. We already know what we should do differently, but the truth is that it just doesn't happen. We are too busy and don't have time to add overwhelming changes into our lives; maybe when things slow down.

Amanda: But what if I were to ask your child whether he would like to:

- Laugh more?
- Feel like he fits in with everyone?
- Have an easier time learning in school?
- Feel calm and happier more often?
- Sleep better at night?
- Have fewer worries?
- Feel like he understands himself, and knows what's going on in his body?

How would your child answer these questions? Would he say sure, how about in six months? Remember, this is not about you. It's about what is best for your child.

It is important to understand that everything comes at a cost. Sure, there is energy and effort that parents will have to put forth in order to make adjustments in their children's lifestyles. But recognize that taking no action also comes at a cost. Think of:

- The sleepless nights you will continue to have, worrying about your child
- The drain you feel each time your child has another reactive situation – at school, at home, at a family party
- The apprehension you feel for how medication side effects affect your child
- The mental anguish you feel when your child is upset and feels like it's their fault

- The deep sadness you experience when your child feels misunderstood and loses confidence

How much mental energy will you exert over the next few months, or even years, feeling anxious or worried, rather than feeling empowered and optimistic because you are discovering how you can help your child right now!?

Mike: Listen, if you're feeling a little turned off at this point, keep reading. We wanted to get your attention on purpose, because the information you are going to uncover about the "deeper why" is so important to the long-term health of your child and your family. We are here to guide you through, step-by-step, so that you can come through the other side armed with your Level 3 Why, have a good sense of *what* needs to happen next, and be ready to implement *how* you can change your child's life.

Amanda: I can't emphasize enough how uplifting this was for us. When you hear about our story, you will see how some of the recommendations for our daughter were things that we understood were not the best solutions for her. We were able to have honest, respectful and helpful conversations with doctors, school administrators, and others about how best to support her recovery and she healed in record time.

Kelly: You bring up an interesting point. If reading this book gives me a chance to feel on the same playing field with all of the experts who give suggestions about my children's well-being, it's a big shift.

Chapter 3

Our Story

Kelly: Tell us a little about your story. How did you become family health experts?

Mike: Love that question, it reminds me of the time I was asked the same thing at a birthday party for a friend's son. My buddy, Jim, had recently learned about my career switch, and asked, "So how did you become a family health expert?" I started into the story about how we have had a total transformation in our family's health, and my daughter Avery runs up to my leg with cake frosting smeared across her face, and vomits all over Jim. Let's just say the conversation didn't go as planned.

The truth is, we know what you're going through if you're worried about a child, because we had our own year from hell. It all started on a Sunday afternoon when our girls were doing homework. Out of the blue, our oldest daughter Julia started having a seizure. It was the first time either one of us had ever seen a seizure. We both felt scared to death.

We didn't know how to handle a seizure or even the slightest idea of what was happening, so I dialed 9-1-1 immediately. By the time the paramedics arrived she had stopped seizing and was resting on the couch. They recommended we take a trip to the emergency room. Amanda had a strong intuitive sense against it, but I insisted we go. How could it hurt, right?

19

To our surprise, the hospital was probably not the right solution for us at the time. As it turns out, Julia was so fearful of the doctors, and the stories she heard of the situation, that she continued to seize every time multiple doctors came into the room to monitor her. The stress on her body was too much. To understand the whole context of the story, we have to give a little background on what had taken place the 48 hours before her first seizure. Julia had been with me at a daddy/daughter group campout weekend. She spent 2 nights staying up until all hours of the night and waking up with the sunrise, snacking on Twizzlers, Doritos and other junk food. Also, she participated in many activities including a pellet gun shooting, riding a huge bungie plunge (which she was scared to do at first) and even a live teen band concert complete with strobe lights. As you will see throughout the book the impact of all of those things caused an overload of stress response which turned her light switch on overdrive. When she woke up Sunday morning at the campout she threw up and slept on the drive home. The last straw was stress about finishing homework in time for school Monday morning, which triggered her first seizure.

Amanda: The crazy part was she was hospitalized for four days, and she had one episode each day, and it always happened when a group of doctors on rounds came in to examine her. We worked with the best pediatric neurologists in the city and ran every test to determine what was going on with our daughter. We were shocked that there didn't seem to be an explanation to what we thought were simple questions like, "Why did she start having seizures? What was causing the seizures? How do we stop them from happening?" The results of her tests were inconclusive, there was nothing in her brain to indicate why they were happening. We were told that sometimes these things just happen in children around her age and hopefully she will grow out of it. The best solution provided was to give her medication. So like any concerned parents, we asked "What's in the medication? What does it do to her body and mind?" Here's where it starts to get scary. The medications had three pages of possible negative side effects. Many required blood test monitoring to ensure that her kidney function wasn't damaged.

However, no one seemed to be addressing the thing that I knew in my heart was part of the issue causing her seizures. It seemed obvious to me that there was a link to her fear when the doctors came into the room and the trigger of each episode. In addition, I knew all of the events from the weekend had to tie to the cause. I asked about the link to her emotions and stimuli, but that is not the area of expertise for neurologists, so it wasn't given much attention.

Kelly: That does seem shocking; it's almost common sense that her emotions had to be tied to her seizures. So what did you do?

Mike: Now we were stuck between a rock and a hard place. Do we do what the doctors suggest, give her medication that could cause long-term harm to her body, while only addressing the symptoms rather than the root cause, or do we look somewhere else for answers? We finally decided it was our top priority to stop the seizures as soon as possible *and* search for a viable long term solution, so she could heal.

Amanda: I felt very uneasy about the long list of negative side effects from the medications, and felt unsettled about the cause of the seizures. My heart knew it had to be related to her emotions and the stress she experienced. This is how our search for the *Level 3 Why* started.

These were without a doubt the most difficult four months of our lives. Julia continued to have seizures, sometimes as many as 10 to 15 in a day. We lived in constant fear about when the next episode was going to happen, because it could become a life or death situation. One day I pulled her up from the bottom of my parent's swimming pool after a seizure. Another time she fell over in her bedroom and cracked her mirror with her head. Every day we were living on eggshells. The crazy thing was that this was our oldest daughter, and we felt like we had to pay such close attention to her all the time that our other three girls, including our two-year-old at the time, weren't getting enough attention.

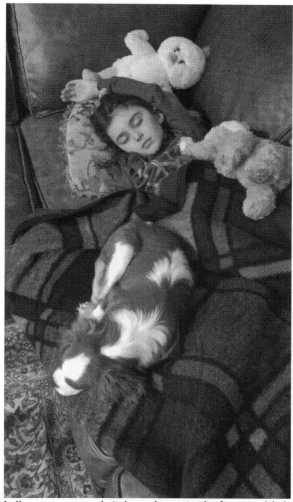

Julia was completely exhausted after multiple
seizures most days.

It was also a rough time for our marriage. Mike and I both felt tremendous guilt; how could this happen, what could we have done better, so she didn't have to face this challenge? Will she have to live like this for the rest of her life? Will she ever be able to drive? We blamed ourselves, we blamed each other, and there were many days when we felt really hopeless about the future. For a while, we were on different pages, and this caused even more tension in our relationship. Mike felt strongly about trying more medication to control her seizures, because they needed to stop for her safety, and I worried about what all of the chemicals were doing to her brain. Especially when we saw our usually sharp, energetic, and vibrant girl change in temperament and confidence. She was eventually taking four different seizure medications at the same time to control her episodes.

Mike: During this time our personal health was under attack, as well. I was having major issues of my own. The only way to really describe it would be extreme anxiety brought on by stress. When our daughter started having seizures, I was working a high-stress job, managing a billion-dollar commodity trading fund at Mesirow Financial. Times were tough, and I would trade through the night, getting two to three hours of sleep, at best. The last thing I needed was additional stress on myself, especially because of my daughter's health. Something worse was bound to happen, and it did.

It started one night when the entire left side of my body went completely numb and I lost all bodily functions. My arm started shaking uncontrollably to the point where my drink was flying everywhere.

That was the beginning of a long miserable year, during which I ended up in the emergency room on numerous occasions, saw many doctors and specialists, and ran every test in the book but ended up with inconclusive explanations for my problems. Finally, after exhausting all western medicine routes I turned to the information Amanda was uncovering about how to help our daughter, and was shocked, because it worked! We were learning how to balance our nervous system in order to heal and maintain health. Our bodies' nervous system has two modes of functioning. We will discuss this more in a later step, but for now just remember there is a sympathetic and a parasympathetic mode. The easiest way to think of it is like a light switch.

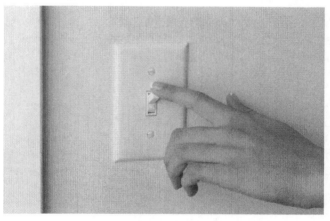

The key to health and happiness is to find balance in your life where some of the hours are spent with your light on and some with it turned off. Just like if you were to leave a light on in your house all the time, it will burn out much faster than if you only turn it on when needed, our bodies' burn out faster too. That is how our health is affected. We will discuss the nervous system in more detail and use the light switch analogy throughout the book to demonstrate how impactful it is.

Amanda: The final piece of the puzzle was the fact that I was suffering from an auto-immune condition called Hashimoto's Thyroiditis that was discovered during my fourth pregnancy. I had spent years trying to get it under control and tried everything from seeing multiple doctors, including MDs, doctors of Osteopathic medicine, going gluten free, and taking many expensive supplements, but nothing was able to turn my condition around until I realized all of the things causing my light switch to be on chronically and started to be intentional about turning it off.

Mike and I have spent tens of thousands of dollars and dedicated years learning about holistic health. You see, I've always had a passion for health. It started in the year 2000, with my career as an AFAA certified fitness instructor and CSCS certified personal trainer. My passion grew, and led me to become an Integrative Nutrition Health Coach through the Institute of Integrative Nutrition, led by my mentor Joshua Rosenthal, one of the pioneers of holistic health. During this training, I studied over 100 different dietary theories.

Mike: Since then, both of us have worked extensively with experts, including Registered Nutritionist Karen Hurd, health advocate Peter Greenlaw, chiropractor Dr. Tommy John, chiropractors Drs. Quintin and Katie Sleigh, therapists Lynn Barrett and Alicia Birong, Life Recalibration coach Allen Vaysberg, and mindset mentor Fabienne Fredrickson, as well as many others.

Amanda: Throughout our journey to heal our own family, we were determined to find answers first-hand. In fact, Monsanto, the largest seller of genetically modified seed (GMOs), invited me to their headquarters in St Louis in 2015 for a tour of their research headquarters and answered my questions directly. Prior to going to Monsanto, I felt very strongly about the dangers of GMOs. However, after spending time learning about the process, my conclusions were shocking. Foods made with GMOs do have a dangerous health potential, but that risk is only problematic for people who eat large amounts of highly processed foods and have compromised immunity which ties back to light switch being on too often.

I was also chosen to be a member of the 2014 Illinois Farm Families City Mom's Program sponsored by the Illinois Farm Bureau. As a member of the program, I spent a year touring various Illinois farms, and learned the latest practices of the dairy, hog, cattle, corn, and soybean farmers. This opportunity provided unparalleled insight into many controversial topics in both organic and conventional farming industries.

Mike: Within one year, we ended up curing our daughter's seizures, my anxiety, and Amanda's auto-immune condition. Three completely different ailments with our knowledge of holistic health, but that wasn't the amazing part. What was truly amazing was that we cured these three ailments using the exact same process.

Amanda: The incredible thing is that we had so many other awesome things we didn't even expect as a result. For example, all four of our daughters gained confidence, we feel closer as a family now than ever before, we spend more time doing things we enjoy and less of things we don't. Everyone has stronger health, Mike lost over 30 pounds, our other daughter Avery's eczema and severe Molluscum Contagiosum cleared up, and Mike was able to eliminate the severe allergies he's had since he was a kid. It is so amazing because all of this happened with zero downside risks!

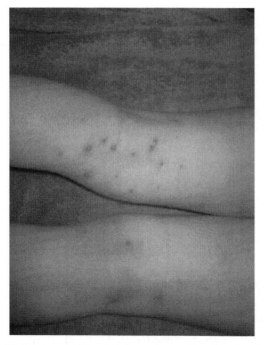

Molluscum Contagiosum on the back of Avery's legs

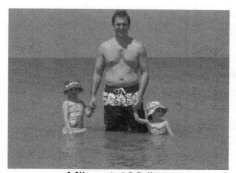

Mike at 193 lbs.

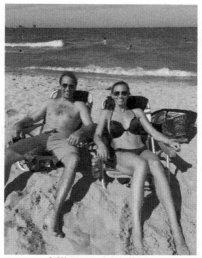

Mike at 160 lbs.

Another thing that played a key role in Julia's recovery was the fact that we found an incredible pediatric neurologist. This doctor was open-minded, and respected the fact that we understood the

Level 3 Why of emotional stress that was affecting our daughter's situation. We were able to work collaboratively with him to create a customized care plan that was best for our daughter. For example, typically a child with her medication regime would receive routine blood tests and EEGs to monitor progress. However, we knew that these things were very stressful for her, and delayed the healing in her brain. Therefore, our doctor carefully explained the risks and respected our decision to forgo the tests because we felt the benefit of information gained was not worth slowing her healing. He also supported her changes in nutrition and activity. As a result, she was able to wean off all four medications and heal in record time. At her last appointment, our doctor said to her with confidence, "Julia you should feel very proud of yourself. I wish you the best, because I'll never see you again!"

We were able to work with school administrators and forego creating an IEP because in our daughter's case, we understood that even though she placed a lot of pressure on herself in an academic environment, if special accommodations for testing, or other scenarios, were provided, she would internally feel more stress because of the distinction from her classmates. When we knew that reducing her stress response was most important for her healing, it was an easy decision.

Mike: We are living proof of the amazing ability of the human body to heal when you give it a chance. We put the pieces of the puzzle together and discovered a deep understanding of how our bodies function, and what they need to work well. We uncovered the dramatic changes in today's society that impact the way we eat, the way we live, and the way we learn; and have found an up-to-date way to optimize health and happiness.

That is how the Hinman Family Health Method was born, and why we have decided to dedicate our lives to this cause. There are so many parents who are looking for answers and are not sure what to believe because of the mountains of conflicting information. Not only that, but often you feel like you are alone and without support when these challenges come up. We understand how overwhelming it can be, so that's why we created the specific 7 Steps you need to create vibrant health and happiness for your family and provide a supportive community to help parents on their journey.

Kelly: Wow, you guys have an amazing story. You have been through a lot and I'm impressed with your extensive research and training to become family health experts.

Chapter 4

New Beginnings

Kelly: It is crazy to hear how one approach can help in such different situations. To be honest, I was wondering where this was going when in the beginning you talked about parents who are concerned about their children, whether they have ADD, allergies, diabetes, or seizures. It seemed like those things are all very different.

Mike: Yes, it is amazing how much overlap there is when it comes to our health. I'm going to toss a crazy idea out and want you to keep it in mind as we discuss the 7 Steps. It's a very provocative claim, so I'll be interested to see what your thoughts are later. What if you have a child with a diagnosis, and I told you the diagnosis doesn't really matter?

Kelly: I'd say you're nuts, of course it matters. A child with a peanut allergy is very different from a child with irritable bowel syndrome. Now I'm really curious to learn more about your approach. Where do you start?

Mike: Before we dive into our Hinman Family Health Method, please understand we do not give any recommendations about medications. In fact, we recognize that there are situations, during an acute phase, when medications provide a great benefit. However, it has been our experiences that in most cases, medications offer short-term relief, but they are not necessary for long-term health.

This is because the role of medication is to alter the chemical balance in your body. Therefore, once a person is able to identify what type of imbalance was causing the problem and then chooses alternative lifestyle choices, they learn how to balance the chemical reactions in their body naturally. We always refer our clients to work with their doctors regarding any adjustments to medications or supplements.

So you may be thinking to yourself, if medication can create the same chemical change in the body as lifestyle changes, wouldn't it be easier to take medication? Perhaps, but please note that the reason lifestyle change is a preferred long-term health strategy is that every medication comes with some unintended consequences. Our bodies are designed to function optimally given the environment they are placed in. Therefore, if a person is experiencing a symptom that is not ideal, the body will find some way to signal that there needs to be a shift in the environment in order to enjoy a different outcome.

When a person forces a chemical shift through medication, but doesn't address the underlying cause, it will continue to be problematic for the body. In addition, medications always affect other areas of the body. For example, many anti-anxiety medications decrease feelings of worry or stress a person feels, but they also diminish feelings of joy, love, and excitement, because the receptors in the brain that are responsible for processing emotions are the same for both positive and negative emotions. These unintended consequences have a way of masking our bodies' natural signals, and then more problems can be created. Statistics prove that people who take medication long-term end up with an increasing number of prescriptions.

Dr. Maya Shetreat-Klein is an integrative pediatric neurologist with a medical degree from Albert Einstein College of Medicine, Board certified in adult and child neurology as well as pediatrics. In her book *The Dirt Cure* she shares concern she sees in her practice about chronic illness that has become the new "normal" for children. She says,

"These kids – maybe even your own kids - go from colic at six weeks, to eczema at six months to chronic ear infections at one year to tubes or a tonsillectomy at three years to an ADD diagnosis at six. Many kids have medication lists that would rival those of senior citizens: steroid cream for eczema; H2 blockers for gastric reflux; antihistamines for allergies; anti-inflammatories for migraines; Miralax for constipation; stimulants for ADHD and learning disabilities; SSRIs for depression; mood stabilizers for anxiety…. sometimes all prescribed at the same time! And more and more kids take insulin for type 1 diabetes or metformin for type 2 diabetes; thyroid medication for hypothyroidism; antiepileptics for seizures; antipsychotics for explosive behavior or anxiety; and steroids or other immune modulators like chemotherapeutics for a wide range of autoimmune diseases that have become shockingly common in children."[3]

This is especially sad because our bodies are capable of finding balance with no negative (only positive) side effects when we make holistic lifestyle changes.

Mike: The final claim is that there is no blame. A challenging situation that is affecting your child or your family is not your fault, or anyone's fault, for that matter. The reality is that whenever you add kids to the equation, there is additional stress, even in a healthy way, on your relationship with your spouse. There are so many unknowns to figure out, plus blending of family traditions. You're stuck figuring out if your parents were geniuses or if what they suggest is ridiculous! This change alone creates a big shift in the relationship between parents. You may have been in a really good spot, and then all of a sudden, you find yourself lost because you prioritize your kid's needs over your own. The guilt of admitting that ever since your kids arrived there are differences between the two of you is too overwhelming, so rather than acknowledging the stress that comes with figuring out how kids fit into YOUR happy, healthy life, you may end up blaming yourself, or each other.

Amanda and I started by blaming ourselves at first, but that quickly escalated to blaming each other. That's when the situation got worse, and things really got ugly in the Hinman household. I would never wish those times upon anyone. As a father, it has always been my responsibility to provide for and protect my family. All of a sudden, I found myself in a situation where the health of my family was breaking down, physically and emotionally, my marriage was on the rocks, and I was not trading well. The last thing I needed to worry about was money. I almost felt relieved when the doctors didn't have answers to my daughter's problems. It basically let me off the hook. It was easier for me to accept the fact that there was nothing we could do, and she was going to take medication, potentially for the rest of her life. Amanda felt differently, and this was really rough for us for a while.

Amanda: It's hard to explain, but as a parent, you may have an intuitive feeling about things sometimes. I knew in my heart that there was something more going on, but I didn't know how to help, so I felt incredibly guilty. I had no idea about all of the factors that can lead to an imbalance in the body, or how to help our daughter, so I felt like a failure as a mom. To make matters worse, because Mike seemed to be accepting that there was nothing else we could do, I started to have less respect for his opinions. This made him feel like I didn't respect how he was taking care of and protecting our daughter. He thought he was protecting her the best he could by increasing her medications. If you are feeling even a fraction of the blame and guilt that we both felt, then our hearts are with you. That is exactly why we are so passionate about sharing this information with you now.

Mike: I can't stress enough that there is no guilt or blame on your end. Everyone knows you would have done anything within your power to stop or reverse the situation for your child. And the proof is the fact that you are reading this book.

The reality is that being a parent is the toughest job on earth, and most of us don't ever take a class or learn how to do it. We just kind of wing it, and learn as we go, based on what our parents did or didn't do. The biggest shift in perspective that I want to share with you is the fact that our world is changing dramatically. Seems obvious, I know. All you have to do is look around and see that there are new, updated versions of phones every six months. There have been such huge shifts in all areas of our lives, and that means if we stick with the same information we had growing up about health and happiness, we are living an outdated way of life. Which one would you rather rely on?

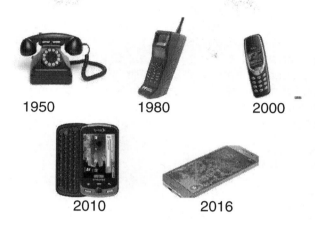

1950   1980   2000

2010   2016

Amanda: Mike is right; this was such an important concept for us to learn about. This is why understanding changes in how we eat, how we live, and how we learn can completely transform our health and happiness. Remember in the introduction, we talked about how the American food supply has changed more in the last 20 years than it had in the prior 200 years? That means that our kids are most likely eating things that didn't even exist when our parents were kids. This impacts **how we eat**. With anything new, there is a learning curve, and we need to know all of the facts about how this new food works in our bodies before we can really understand the impact it has.

The second change affecting **how we live** is the fact that an average person today takes in more information through their senses in one 24-hour period than our parents did in an entire year when they were kids. That means that our children are literally processing more information in one year than our great-grandparents did in their entire life. Stop and think about that! You will learn how this much stimuli dramatically affect the way our bodies function and how we live. One example is the increasing number of pixels on your TV screen, tablet or phone. Sure, the higher pixel count provides a sharper image, but it also means more work for our brains to sift through and process.

Mike: The third change that affects **how we learn** is the dramatic change in education. With increasing globalization and economic pressure, our country's laws have changed the public academic environment. There are more standardized tests, more stringent metrics of academic success and overall more pressure for both teachers and students. In addition, many kids today participate in more structured sports practices, music lessons or other extracurricular activities. This leaves less time for unstructured creativity in our children's lives. We will share how the lack of creativity can lead to chronic negative stress, which is very detrimental to health.

So what do all of these changes mean? They simply mean that we have to learn what new information is helpful to live a healthy and happy lifestyle in the 21st century. The great thing is that there is so much we are learning now about how the human body functions and what things affect our health. It's a double-edged sword, though, because there is a TON of information and it becomes overwhelming. Add to it the fact that a lot of information is conflicting and you would rather toss up your hands and forget about it.

Amanda: That is why we provide a proven 7-Step proprietary system that is the exact process you need to guide your child to health. We have been in your shoes before, and spent thousands of dollars and over ten years becoming holistic health parenting experts. We designed a comprehensive and logical approach that works. The Hinman Family Health Method will enable you to uncover the *why*, *what,* and *how* of helping your child live his best life. What makes our method unique is that we utilize a bio-individual approach that focuses on listening to your body. Each person is unique and there are literally thousands of different combinations that work for different people. We teach you how to listen to your body's signals and guide your children to do it too, rather than providing a cookie-cutter plan for everyone.

Mike: I mentioned before we have cut through the crap and will present you with the facts so you can make an informed choice of what is right for your family. We are committed to providing you with as much helpful information as possible, including links to many other valuable resources. After reading this book you are guaranteed to improve the long-term health and happiness of everyone in your family!

Kelly: First of all, thank you for acknowledging all the parents reading this book. It feels really good to start off from a place of releasing blame. I'm ready to learn how to help my kids.

Chapter 5

SEE How You Prioritize Health

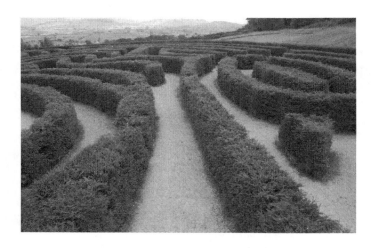

Kelly: Let's get started. What is the first step in the Hinman Family Health Method?

Amanda: The first step is "SEE How You Prioritize Health." As Steven Covey, author of *The 7 Habits of Highly Effective People*,[4] says, "You can't hit a target you can't see." It is so obvious, but we often overlook the benefit of stopping to SEE where we are today and then planning for the future. How are you currently prioritizing health? Are Mom and Dad on the same page? As you can tell from our story, we definitely weren't for a while. You have to know where you are today before you begin to SEE what vibrant health and happiness means to your family in the future.

Mike: Yeah, Amanda said you have to see if you both are on the same page. I cannot emphasize this enough. Think of it like this: Imagine that you are learning to water ski. Amanda and I grew up water skiing on Lake Tichigan in Wisconsin. We would always look forward to skiing, either first thing in the morning or after dinner, because the water was smooth as glass. It's awesome skiing in these conditions; you can see where you're going and navigate very easily from side to side. You can really rip it up. However, try to ski in the middle of Saturday afternoon on the Fourth of July weekend…it's insane! The waters are rough and choppy, and it's no fun. You can feel yourself tighten up and struggle while dodging wakes from other boats and jet skis. This is what it is like for children when parents are not on the same page and send mixed messages. Is it any wonder that your kids don't know what to pay attention to or which direction to go if you are creating an environment of choppy water?

We are going to share our <u>SEE How You Prioritize Health Quiz</u> and find out if both parents are in sync with the messages they provide for the family. Answer the following questions. One column is for Mom and the other for Dad. Ideally, each parent will answer the questions for him or herself, but it is possible to have one parent complete both sides. Write a number for each question on a scale from 1 to 10 for how you currently prioritize this in your family's life. 1 means not at all and 10 means yes, absolutely!

SEE How You Prioritize Health Quiz	Dad	Mom
How do you show up every day to support your child's best nutrition for health?		
Do you spend time learning to understand how your child feels loved in their own unique way?		
How much do you prioritize the important of downtime for your family and child?		
Do you create time for your family to be active together in a fun way?		
Do you believe that it is possible for your child to heal from their allergy, anxiety, emotional disorder or physical situation?		
Are you ok with allowing your child to express their emotions, even when they are intense?		

Kelly: This is interesting. I can already see how my husband and I are different on many of these things. So what does this information tell us?

Understanding your Self-Assessment

Mike: Now that you have an idea of what both parents think about different areas of health, let's talk about what we can learn from this. First, compare the numbers you chose for your answers to each question and those of your partner. Each time the two numbers were within a point of each other, tally one point for that column. This is your consistency score. The highest possible total would be 6 points, if you and your partner were within one point of each other for every question. This consistency number is very important.

Consistency Score _____

If your consistency score is 5 or 6, congrats! You are doing a fantastic job of creating smooth waters for your family. It is very helpful for your children to know where they stand and to see what is modeled in front of them as they make decisions for themselves.

If your score is 3 or 4, you are off to a great start. There are many things that Mom and Dad see eye-to-eye on, and this means you probably have many of the same values. There are a couple of areas that you could benefit from taking a closer look at and discovering what the family priorities are. By coming together on the same page even more, you have an opportunity to create a lasting impact on your family's health.

If your consistency score is 2 or less, then this is definitely creating challenges for your children. It is very difficult to see where to go and what to prioritize when an environment is filled with choppy waters. Don't worry, we will continue to provide you with strategies, best practices, and tools, so that both Mom and Dad can take a step in a more consistent direction.

Amanda: Next take an average of Mom and Dad's scores for each question and then add up the total of the average scores. This gives your health score.

Health Score_____

If this total score is 48 or above, the two of you are doing a fantastic job of supporting your child's health, as well as your own. You have a deep understanding of the many areas that contribute to a person's overall health and wellness and you can keep on rocking!

If your score is between 30 and 47, that's good. There are many things that you are doing well, and this has been of huge benefit to your kids. In fact, you have probably already spent time and energy focusing on health, and we have more inspiration, tools, and strategies to help you continue the journey.

If the total was less than 30, no sweat! Remember, as we said, seeing where you are currently is the most important first step. Now you are aware that there are many areas you can learn about to support your child's health. You are here today and that is HUGE! You are in the right place to find out exactly how you can create the type of health and happiness that you want for your child and family.

Mike: Something that is often surprising is that having a low consistency score is usually more detrimental to your child's well-being than having a low health score. This was the case for our family. Even though Amanda was aware of many things that contribute to great health, like eating well and staying active, we were very inconsistent with our messages to the kids. That created a lot of chaos, and today I believe it played a large role in the development of Julia's seizures.

Amanda: It's really amazing, because obviously we realize parents aren't going to always agree on everything, but simply taking the time to discuss how you feel and why opens the door for the two of you to figure out what works best for your family.

Another step that is really helpful during Step 1 of the Hinman Family Health Method is for parents to learn more about themselves and each other. We share information about the DISC behavior styles that were developed by Harvard-educated psychologist Dr. William Moulton Marston. These four behavior styles are Dominant, Influencer, Steady Relater, and Compliance Thinker. When you know what behavior type both you and your partner have, it is easier to communicate and understand each other.

After you have a clear starting point of where you are today, it's time to think about what you want for your family in the future. Sometimes, people find it hard to create a vision or goal for what their life would be in one year, five years, ten years, etc. My dear friend Bailey Frumen, who is a lifestyle design coach and psychotherapist, uses a great tool with her clients. She has them work through an *Ideal Day Visualization*. This is where you take the time to close your eyes, breathe deeply, relax, and then imagine step by step what waking up on your perfect day would feel like. Think about where you are, who is with you, what smells are around you, what you are doing, and so on? The goal is to be as specific as possible and notice what comes up. This is a great way to get your creative juices flowing and come up with a vision for your family's future.

There are two important steps to creating a memorable vision:

1) Make it specific

2) Attach emotion to the outcome

Let's use an analogy of taking a road trip to California. If I were to get into a car and simply drive west heading to California, my destination is very ambiguous. Am I heading toward San Francisco or San Diego?

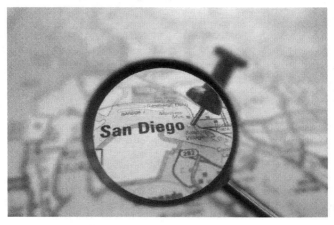

Why am I going? How will I feel when I get there? All of these things affect how I feel and my motivation for going. If I'm looking forward to relaxing on the beach, I'm likely to endure the long car ride, but if I'm going to a work seminar that I dread, it will feel like a hassle. It's a lot easier and more efficient to navigate when I am specific in my vision and recognize the value of why I am traveling in the first place.

Now it's time to write out what your healthy and happy family life will be like in one year, five years, and ten years. We suggest you pause now, and you click this link www.hinmans/familyvison to hear a guided meditation and download a worksheet to support the creation your own one-year, five-year and ten-year vision for your family. Here is a little room for notes to get you started:

One year from now our healthy and happy family life looks like

_____

_____

_____

_____

Five years from now our healthy and happy family life looks like

_____

_____

_____

_____

Ten years from now our healthy and happy family life looks like

_____

_____

_____

_____

After you complete this process, the results of working together to **SEE How You Prioritize Health** are:

- A specific, unified vision of what a healthy and happy family life looks like for you (We've all heard the saying the family that eats together, stays together, but we like to say the couple that thinks together, sleeps together!)

- Clarity on what things your family wants to spend more time/energy on, and what you would like to spend less time/energy on

- Improved time management as a result of that clarity

Kelly: You bring up an interesting topic that I never tied to health before, and that's time management. I hate to admit how much time I spend on things that I don't really care about or that don't make me happy on a daily basis. I had never thought about how it can affect my health or my child's health. This has me thinking about Dylan. I'm sure part of the reason he loves his sports so much is because it's fun and school is boring to him.

Mike: For sure, when you end up spending the majority hours in your day feeling obligated to do everything, rather than grateful to do it, you end up with a lot of stress. I'm a little too familiar with just how much stress can kill you!

Also, I am happy to share we have created a **Bonus Resource Guide** which provides supplemental material for all of the information listed in this book. This guide provides links to videos, worksheets, articles, and suggested books mentioned throughout. We will provide a short summary of what information you can find after each step, so it is easy to find what you are looking for. Download your free Bonus Resource Guide here: **www.hinmans/BonusRG.com**.

Step 1 – SEE How You Prioritize Health – Bonus Resource Guide includes:

- SEE How You Prioritize Health Quiz PDF

- Understanding Your Assessment PDF

- Family Vision Guided Audio/PDF

- Video about DISC behavioral styles.

Chapter 6

FEED Your Body Well

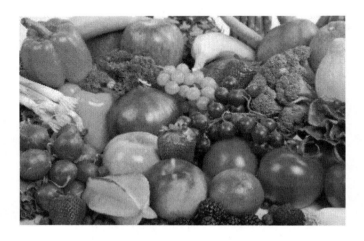

Kelly: Ok, so now that I'm clear on where my family life is today and what direction we want to move towards, what's next?

Amanda: The next step to think about is how you nourish your body. Did you know that all of the cells in our bodies are constantly regenerating? In other words, our bodies are being rebuilt all the time. The average person has an entirely new skeletal system every seven years, new intestinal lining in six months, etc. Your organs, tissues, and muscles are constantly changing, because new cells replace the old ones. Each new cell is created from the food we put into our bodies. Our food is literally the building blocks of our bodies. Another way to think about it is food is *information* for our bodies, quite literally it is the *input* that *forms* our physical bodies.

Change 1 – How We Eat

Another thing that we mentioned before is the fact that the American food supply is so dramatically different today. In other words, the foods that most people eat today are not the same as what our parents and grandparents ate. This is particularly true for any packaged foods. All you have to do is turn over the box and look at the ingredient label. Notice how many of the ingredients are words you don't even recognize? We don't know what those ingredients are, and neither do our bodies. Many people are eating things that their bodies can't ever use to make new cells. It's no wonder people are always feeling hungry and having cravings. They don't feel satisfied because their bodies are not getting the materials to make new parts! In addition, these unrecognizable ingredients are treated like invaders in our bodies which turn our light switch on. Just like if a child thinks they heard a monster in their closet, now their eats are tuned in to every squeak and hum in the house, his body goes into protection mode when it is bombarded with unrecognizable invaders and causes a response. For many kids the response is an allergic reaction.

Mike: Listen, we realize that for many people, eating well is the most challenging part, and it's mostly because there is SO much information, and a lot of it is conflicting, about what is the best way to eat. Is animal protein good for you, or is it better to be vegetarian? Is a low-carb Paleo diet the answer, or do you just need to eliminate gluten?

It shouldn't be this difficult to eat well. As a society, we have lost touch with our instincts to know what works well for our bodies and what doesn't. Think of it this way, does a deer in the forest ever stop to consider how many carbs are in the leaves or what the appropriate serving size of nuts is? Obviously, the answer is no. All animals are in tune with their natural instincts about what, when and how much to eat. Ever notice how your dog doesn't eat when he's not feeling well?

Our approach is one that simplifies learning how to feed your body well. We teach the concept of bio-individuality, meaning that there is no one perfect way to eat for everyone. What is one person's food can be another's poison.

Amanda: The number one question we hear from parents is "How do I get my kids to eat better?" It seems that no matter how hard we try, they just won't eat many veggies, meats, etc. The reality is that it's not a simple answer. You can't simply make your kids eat different foods; you could try, but that raises a whole host of other issues, so learn from my mistake and don't do it!

Here's a chance for me to get real and tell you that for many years I was the queen of food policing in our house. My girls still have vivid memories of me monitoring their sugar intake at family parties and commenting on how we should eat organic only. It's still really hard for me to let go of control when I feel like my girls are eating something that's bad for them. Sometimes it feels like I know too much and life would be easier if I didn't! Would you let your child open up a bottle of bleach and drink it? Of course not, but because so many of the effects of poor nutrition don't appear until days, months, or even years later, it's hard for kids to understand the urgency.

By continuing through the steps in this book you will uncover the Level 3 Why of a child is a picky eater. You will understand that there is a link to other areas in his life. Nothing happens in isolation. For example, nine-year-old Tommy craves sugar frequently. In fact, if it were up to him, he would probably be happy to live on pasta, Doritos, and cookies for the rest of his life. It's a battle to try and get him to eat broccoli, beans, pork chops, or anything for dinner besides chicken tenders and mac-n-cheese. The deeper reason why Tommy has such strong cravings for sugar could be because his light switch is turned on too much. When his body is in light switch on mode, it is burning high amounts of glucose (sugar). In other words, Tommy's body is simply signaling to him that he needs to continually restore his blood glucose levels, because that's what the environment is demanding. As long as there is no shift made in his nervous system, he will never have the willpower to change his eating habits. The same is true for adults. We tend to be able to "eat well" for a little longer than kids, maybe long enough to do a two-week cleanse or something, but if we don't ever look deeper and understand why our body is signaling what it is, then we will fall off the wagon too.

Kelly: This is interesting. Kate is a really picky eater, and basically, the only thing she likes to eat is bread, cereal, or some other sweet treat. I never thought about her body burning tons of sugar because of how her nervous system is working.

You mean to tell me this could change if her nervous system adjusts?

Amanda: Yes, it can and will change. Now, to be fair, our bodies are designed to enjoy the taste of sugar and we will talk more about why later, but excessive cravings will change. Sugar cravings played a big role in the development of my auto-immune condition. My routine consisted of eating eggs or smoothie for breakfast, salads for lunch, and a healthy dinner of veggies and meat. But after the kids were in bed I would crave sugar like crazy and eagerly bake up a fresh batch of chocolate chip cookies topped with a big dollop of buttercream frosting and sit on the couch to watch Scandal. I couldn't understand why my cravings were so controlling. It wasn't until I understood the impact of my nervous system and shifted other things around in my life that it changed.

Another thing that's important for families is convenience. Parents are busy, and have limited time for food preparation. So it's important to understand what the key nutrients each body needs to work well are. We want to work smarter, not harder, right? If you focus your energy on providing those things, you'll learn quick and easy ways to add real foods into your family's life. When your child's body is being filled up with what it needs to work well their emotions stabilize and they don't drive you crazy constantly snacking without ever eating meals.

Mike: The key nutrients for all humans are proteins, fiber, vitamins, minerals, and essential fats. Perhaps the single most impactful change for someone challenged by allergies, anxiety, or difficulty concentrating is increasing soluble fiber.

The best source of soluble fiber is legumes or beans. The reason this is so helpful is because fiber works with your liver to detoxify your blood and is able to pull toxins, allergens, and excess hormones out of your body in the form of a bowel movement. Yes, it's true we are just getting to know each other, and already I'm talking about poop! You've heard it from Dr. Oz; your poop is one the best barometers of what is going on inside your body!

So one easy strategy to help your child today is to add beans to their food. Black beans, kidney beans, garbanzo, cannellini, lima, you name it. All are good!

Amanda: Yeah, Mike is right. This is probably the biggest shift that our clients see in their lives. Once you understand how the liver works, and the fact that all of your body's garbage (excess hormones, toxins, and metabolic waste) are just waiting to get to the toilet, but the exit strategy doesn't happen if you don't have enough fiber in your diet; it is life changing. Did you know that for most Americans, up to 95% of their waste gets dumped right back into the blood stream? This is at the heart of so many chronic conditions. When all of our body's garbage is put right back into our blood, it triggers so many unintended consequences, such as allergies, excess hormones that lead to anxiety, inflammation, and inability to concentrate just to name a few. Registered Nutritionist Karen Hurd was the person that taught us about the importance of detoxifying our blood using beans. We credit a large portion of our family's healing – from Julia's seizures, to Mike's anxiety and allergies, Avery's Molluscum Contagiosum, and my Hashimoto's – to the cleaning of our blood supply and changes in our biochemistry.

Let me point out, for some people who are challenged with ulcerative colitis, Crohn's disease, or other digestive distress, it is often recommended that they eliminate fiber from their diets, because it is irritating to the digestive system. It is true that eliminating fiber, and all other inflammatory foods, for a short time during an acute flare-up is important to allow the intestinal lining to heal. However, we stress how important it is to reintroduce fiber into the diet as a long-term health strategy once the flare up has receded. This is because fiber is essential to clean our blood supply and detoxify the body. It is one of the keys to maintaining balance and heal permanently from those types of conditions.

Families that have been faced with this type of challenge are always shocked to learn about Leo, who was diagnosed with Crohn's disease at age two. He was originally told he would have to learn to use steroid medication to manage the disease for the rest of his life and avoid high fiber foods. Within a year, he completely healed the Crohn's disease, is medication free, and his entire family eats beans every day, because they understand how important fiber is to maintaining strong health.

Mike: Listen, we understand this is a lot of information and probably stuff you have never heard of before, but remember this is the tip of the iceberg here. Fiber is only one of the essential nutrients our bodies need to work well. Other things, like protein, vitamins, minerals, and essential fats are important, too. In fact, proteins are the building blocks of every cell in your body.

Earlier you learned that our bodies are constantly regenerating, so they need protein every day. According to Karen Hurd, it is important to have adequate sources of protein that are both complete and efficient. There are only five sources that are both, and by eating protein sources that may not be efficient the body is forced to work much harder to build new cells and this results in extraordinary amounts of metabolic waste, which puts a large burden on the liver to detoxify and increases a person's need for fiber. The five sources of complete and efficient proteins are:

- Meat
- Poultry
- Eggs
- Fish
- Seafood

Another essential category of nutrients is minerals. Minerals are like the spark plugs for your body, because you need certain ones in order to make chemical reactions happen so things can run smoothly. In fact, world-renowned health advocate and author Peter Greenlaw shares how important minerals are for healthy brain function. He was the guest speaker at the 2014 and 2015 Autism One Conferences because of his in-depth knowledge about the importance of minerals in improving mental imbalances. Minerals are found in soil, so the best way to increase your child's mineral intake is to eat real foods that are grown in soil or from animals that eat foods grown in soil. Foods high in minerals include legumes (beans), cheeses, meats, vegetables, fruits, and whole grains.

Did you know that what you eat affects your brain?

Kelly: I'm glad you mentioned this because I've read some information about a connection between gut health and brain health. Can you talk a little more about that, and what we need to know to have a healthy gut?

Amanda: Absolutely. Hidden in the walls of the digestive system is the enteric nervous system (ENS), which is called a "second brain". The ENS is two thin layers of more than 100 million nerve cells, and it contains more nerve endings than your brain. "Its main role is controlling digestion, from swallowing, to the release of enzymes that break down food, to the control of blood flow that helps with nutrient absorption, to elimination," explains Jay Pasricha, M.D., director of the Johns Hopkins Center for Neurogastroenterology. "The enteric nervous system doesn't seem capable of thought as we know it, but it communicates back and forth with our big brain – with profound results." [5]

Here is an analogy to simplify the role of our second brain. Think of our second brain like a UPS distribution hub. Mail, packages, and boxes enter the hub, are sorted, grouped, and then delivered to different addresses. This is similar to how our food enters the digestive tract, where the second brain breaks it down into nutrients, sorts the nutrients, and delivers them to cells in our bodies, including in our brains, so they can function properly. Just as the UPS distribution hub needs to have proficient workers to accomplish all of the steps in delivering mail, our second brain needs some good helpers, too. The good helpers in our body are probiotics, which are microscopic organisms and other bacteria that assist the second brain in breaking down and sorting the nutrients.

Eating foods that contain a lot of chemicals and unrecognizable things is like sending mail and packages to the UPS distribution center with no addresses on them. When our bodies can't recognize food, it doesn't know what to do with it. The more processed and chemicalized food a person eats; the more confusion it creates. Also, eating foods that are high in sugars and artificial sweeteners destroys healthy probiotics in our gut and instead provide pathogenic, or detrimental, bacteria. Think of it like having a bunch of irresponsible workers, who sat around on break all day at the UPS hub. The best way to maintain a balance of healthy probiotics is to eat real foods that contain complex carbohydrates and short-chain fatty acids (STFAs), because they serve as the perfect prebiotic, or food, for probiotics. Back to the UPS analogy, I bet you would have a bunch of happy, productive workers if a tasty lunch were provided each day!

The takeaway from all of this information about second brain and probiotics is the food that our kids eat has a huge impact on how everything inside their bodies function. It affects everything from the skin cells in an allergic reaction of hives, to liver function when it can't detoxify the body of excess hormones which cause anxiety, to brain function when a child has difficulty maintaining focus.

Kelly: I like the UPS analogy. It makes it easy to understand that my focus for my family is to eat real foods because then it's like sending mail with addresses to UPS and providing lunch to have happy workers! What kinds of foods will help maintain healthy probiotic balance?

Amanda: This is an easy one, because there are so many! Any type of legume or bean is a great source of complex carbohydrate that also contains STFAs. Also, whole grains such as quinoa, millet, barley, buckwheat, corn, and rice contain complex carbohydrates. Finally, starchy vegetables like sweet potatoes, red potatoes, beets, radishes, peppers, peas, turnips, and parsnips are great too. Perhaps the best source of probiotics is naturally fermented foods like sauerkraut, yogurt, or kimchi. Fermented recipes are fun to make with your kids too! One of our favorites is a simple dilly carrot recipe from Tamara Mannelly from OhLardy.com.

These tangy carrots make a great after school snack, topping for salads, or a quick side dish to serve with dinner. The process of lacto-fermentation, leaving them at room temperature for four to seven days, creates beneficial enzymes, B-vitamins, and various strains of probiotics. These carrots are even healthier than regular carrots, and they taste great too!

Ingredients

- 5 to 7 carrots, peeled and cut into sticks (or bag of baby carrots)
- 1 tsp. sea salt
- 1 Tbsp. fresh dill (or more if you like)
- 3 to 4 cloves of garlic, quartered
- filtered water

Instructions

1. Place your ingredients in a quart-sized Mason jar and fill to within one inch of the top with filtered water.

2. Cover and ferment on your counter for 4 to 7 days.

3. Refrigerate to stop the fermentation process and enjoy!

Kelly: Wow, it sounds so easy! Thanks for the recipe.

Mike: You're welcome, and it is easy. Another thing I want to point out is that Amanda and I don't feel like it is our job to give you a huge list of all the things your child shouldn't eat. Let's face it, you already know what you could change about the way you or your child eats, so it doesn't provide any value to you for us to create a "Do Not Eat" list. Instead of focusing on how deprived your child might feel by cutting things out of his diet, we would rather provide value by teaching you what things are so IMPORTANT for your family to eat, so that everyone's body can work well and make great parts. The truth of the matter is that children learn more by what you do than by what you say. So, a big part of living healthy or healing for your child takes place when parents embrace eating more real foods themselves.

We don't talk about counting calories or fat grams because when you eat real foods in their natural state, you don't ever have to worry about all the other stuff. Nature already did the calculations, and put the right amount of calories, fat, fiber, and so on, and in the perfect blend. When you listen to your body, notice how different balances of foods make you feel, and understand the role of the key nutrients, you will know how to make your own adjustments throughout life to feel your best. By the time you eat all of the important nutrients to feel good, there really isn't that much room left for the crappy stuff.

In fact, when I first changed my eating habits I was constantly eating. Not once did I count a calorie or fat gram. Whenever I was hungry, I just ate. The amazing part was that even though I was constantly shoving food in my face, as long as I focused on putting foods that mattered into my mouth, I still lost weight. Over time, my taste buds even changed, and today I prefer the healthy option over my old go-to, a beef sandwich and cheese fries from Portillo's.

Amanda: Yes, Mike is right. We encourage you to crowd out the highly processed, "chemicalized" food by adding in the good stuff. Going back to the top question we receive: "How do I get my kids to eat better?" Our recommendation is to focus on the good stuff first. No one wants to hear what they can't have or how bad something they enjoy is for them. It's important to talk about what the benefit is to your kids, in terms they understand, when they eat real foods. Point out connections to food in their daily lives. For example, a high score on a math test because they ate avocado for lunch, which helped their brain focus; or scoring a goal in soccer because they ate broccoli, which builds strong muscles. The more clearly parents communicate the connection to food, the more open children become.

Realize that this takes time. Patience is important, because until a shift in the nervous system happens, it's fighting an uphill battle. There is nothing wrong with their cravings, however, willpower alone cannot overcome thousands of years of physiological evolution. It is how are bodies are designed. Some other changes are needed to shift the environment inside their body. That is why a holistic approach is crucial, and we provide 7 Steps in the Hinman Family Health Method.

Remember, **Change 1 – How We Eat** is affected by our food supply. By focusing on eating real foods in their natural state, your family will be eating foods that promote health. A good rule of thumb is if your grandmother wouldn't recognize it, you shouldn't eat it.

To sum it up, we encourage parents to go through three phases of learning how to FEED their families.

1. Pay attention to what you and your child are eating, and focus on eating as many real foods as possible.

2. Be intentional about including all of the essential ingredients everyone's body needs to work well and make good parts.

3. Notice how the foods make you feel and what you see in your child's life, too.

It all boils down to just **paying attention** to what you are eating. As far as picky eaters, you would be surprised at how resilient kids are, once they learn what makes them feel good and what doesn't. Usually, it's just that the connection between food and mood has never been brought to their attention before. When you approach feeding yourself well with this mindset, you discover many benefits, including:

- More awareness about the choices and situations in your current life that may be negatively affecting your child's health.

- A deeper understanding of how our bodies work and what things are important to fuel them.

- A sense of empowerment because now you understand how you can drastically improve your child's health, as well as your own.

Kelly: It's interesting to me that you talk about food – and I've got to be honest, at first I kind of cringed, because I already know I should eat better. The messages to eat healthy are all around us, yet I tune them out most of the time, because I never had anyone share the perspective that my body and my kid's bodies are designed to crave sugar sometimes, and it's really up to me to find out what works best with my body. I didn't realize that our bodies are literally being built with food that we eat. I always assumed you're born with what you're born with, and there's not much you can do to change it.

Mike: I know what you mean; it's pretty life-changing. I like cars, and for me it's like, would I rather drive an Aston Martin with a high-performance engine that corners on rails, or an old beater? I had to ask myself, what kind of parts am I making?

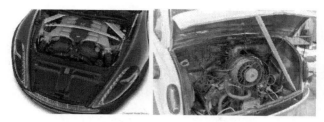

It's the same with your body and your child's too. Once you know what kind of parts you want to build, it is a lot easier to choose real foods over the artificial stuff. And when you become aware of how much better you actually feel, you'll never want to go back.

Kelly: You're giving me a lot to think about, but yet, it seems like common sense.

Mike: Step 2 – FEED Your Body Well – Bonus Resource Guide includes:

- Video with Registered Nutritionist Karen Hurd discussing the important of fiber

- Video with Registered Nutritionist Karen Hurd discussing protein

- Video with Autism One Speaker Peter Greenlaw discussing the importance of minerals

- Article about Amanda's first-hand experience touring Monsanto Research and Development Headquarters

- Video with Tamara Mannelly demonstrating how to make fermented recipe.

Download here: www.hinmans/BonusRG.com.

Chapter 7

LOVE (and Respect) Your Family Unconditionally

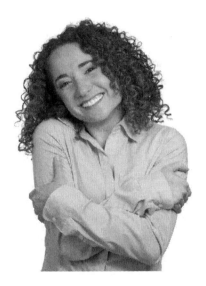

Kelly: Now that I have a vision of what a healthy and happy family looks like in my life, and I'm beginning to understand how important it is to just eat real food, what's next?

Amanda: The next step is being thoughtful about how to LOVE (and respect) your family unconditionally. Is this a picture of how you greet yourself every morning? If not, maybe it should be, according to Allen Vaysberg, author of the book *A New Love Triangle: Your practical guide to a love-filled life!* [6] Of course, anyone reading this book loves his or her family; that's why you're here, but have you ever thought about how much you love yourself?

Probably not; it feels kind of unusual – even selfish. This is not something that is typically taught or talked about. How does the amount that a parent loves himself have anything to do with his child? What if it is at the heart of the matter? Allen shares how this is the most critical first step for everyone. In an airplane, parents are directed to put on their own oxygen masks first, before assisting a child; similarly, we must learn to love and accept ourselves before we can completely love and accept anyone else. Each person has to fill their own cup before they can give to anyone else.

One of our clients, Maria, felt guilty at first prioritizing time for her own self-care. She didn't have time because her life was busy. She worked full time, had three kids active in different things, and wanted to spend time with her husband. I asked her, "Do you want Victoria to feel the same way you do when she is your age?" Maria shared that this was a life-changing moment for her. Once she thought of her daughter feeling what she felt, everything shifted. She realized how important it is to teach her daughter about self-love by being an example and loving herself first.

Mike: At first this was really uncomfortable for me. I thought, of course I love myself. I don't even know how this relates to my daughter's seizures or anything else. But then, when I stopped to take a deeper look at what I love about myself, it was hard to answer. It's much easier to think of things I want to change or improve upon. Self-love is something that each person must figure out for himself.

I'm the type of person who thinks about pleasing others first and foremost. For example, whenever we host a party, I'm always thinking about what foods my guests enjoy the most or raved about at our last party, and I then try to accommodate those needs. I'm always the last one to eat and sometimes that means I get what's left over. To take it a step farther, I always put my kids' needs before my own. That is especially true when it comes to dinner. The kids go for their favorites first, and if it means asking for what's on Daddy's plate, I usually give it to them, and I'm left with their extra Brussels sprouts. What I discovered was that for me, this type of generosity is a type of self-love because I am happiest when I can do something to make others feel good. However, if having a plate of food that I enjoyed made me happiest, these choices would be the opposite of self-love.

Most of us have no problem internally pointing out our flaws rather than feeling patient and accepting of ourselves, although what we show on the outside may be very different. In fact, we usually think things about ourselves that we would never say to a friend. Any type of negative mental chatter or criticism is yet another trigger that turns our light switch on. When a person is able to increase their self-love it is easier to turn the light switch off and find balance.

In addition, if you don't love yourself and accept the mistakes that you inevitably make, it becomes harder to accept mistakes of others. An example for me is when I used to flip out if my daughter spilled milk on the floor. My reaction was intense, and when I stopped to think about why, it was because I felt that she should be more careful. I knew that if I had spilled the milk, I would have berated myself, so it's like my instinct just kicked in to yell before I could filter and accept that it's not a big deal, whoever spilled it. I'm not going to lie; these things still happen, but I'm working on my reactions to myself and others all the time.

Change 3 – How We Learn

Amanda: As parents the things that drive us crazy about our kids are things about which we are self-critical. One example for me is my daughter Isabel's stride and walking with flat feet. I used to always point it out and ask her if she remembered to stretch. I had flat feet as a kid, and am really aware of it. The more accepting of myself I become, the easier it is to keep comments to myself and show unconditional love to her. It's not like my comments changed her gait. Once again, leading by example is the best way for your child to learn to love and accept herself.

This is a great opportunity to have an impact how our kids learn. When we talked about three areas of life that drive health and happiness, one of them was how we learn. Allen shares a great strategy to begin to increase the amount of self-love you feel. Start by taking a piece of paper and write at least one thing that you LOVE about yourself. Keep this paper by your bed, or in another convenient place, and add one thing to the list each day. As you add to your list, remember to look back and read all of the previous things you noted and appreciate the gifts you provide to those around you.

Kelly: This is an interesting perspective. Not where I thought you were going with this step, but I can see how the way you feel about yourself impacts how you treat others. But it still feels weird to think I just have to love myself more and then my kids will feel more confident. This is something I'm going to start to pay attention to and see how it affects our family. Is there anything else you recommend that is more directly tied to loving your child?

Amanda: Yes, learning to love yourself is only part of the process. It's also important to learn if your love and respect are being recognized by other people in your family.

As you said, Kelly, everyone is unique. We interpret things differently – the way we feel, what we enjoy doing – and these differences apply to how we feel loved too.

Have you ever talked with your partner about something, and then felt speechless afterward, when you realized he just didn't get it?

Kelly: Yes, it drives me crazy!

Amanda: Of course, we all have. This same miscommunication happens with love and respect. We do our best to show love to someone but they just don't see it. Or, even worse, they misunderstood it and reacted negatively.

To be honest, I used to totally miss the boat on this with my youngest daughter, Taylor. I like to be very active and involved in different things. To me, signing her up for a dance and gymnastics class was my way of showing her how much I loved her. I felt that I was investing time and money for her to have a fun experience. But she didn't want to do those things. In fact, she never asked to take those classes; I just assumed that she would enjoy them. The reality was that she was feeling pressured into doing something that wasn't interesting to her at that time. So instead of feeling my love, Taylor felt that she wasn't accepted for who she was and what she enjoyed doing with her time.

The amazing thing was that once I realized this, and pulled out of the classes, there were no longer battles to get her to class on time, and within six months she was ready and asked to take gymnastics on her own. Then she happily went to class and we didn't stress about being late. As it turns out, dance still isn't her thing.

Kelly: I know exactly what you mean. Looking back on it now, I can see how different my son and daughter are. Dylan is like me, and wants to be involved in everything. He plays soccer, basketball, baseball, is in Cub Scouts, and seems to love it all. But I guess I didn't think about how Kate is different from us. It takes forever for her to get ready and in the car for dance and soccer. Many times, she freaks out about putting on her leotard or ends up in tears during the soccer game. I knew she was sensitive, but didn't really stop to think that maybe she doesn't love doing these things. She is happiest when she is at home coloring, or when we play make-believe together.

Amanda: Yeah, it's pretty humbling to see that our kids give us signals all the time about what they love and what they don't, but sometimes we are so busy with our own agenda that we miss it.

Kelly: So is there anything else parents can do besides look for behaviors from their kids about what they love and what they don't?

Mike: Watching your kids' behaviors is a great place to start. There are also great tools to find out how everyone in your family recognizes love. This is SO important because many times, one person is spending a lot of effort trying to show love, but it is not recognized. That person starts to feel rejected, and the other person feels misunderstood. The key to feeling loved is to feel understood!

Gary D. Chapman, author of *Five Love Languages*,[7] talks about five different ways people recognize love. Most people naturally show love in their own language, but once you learn how others feel love, a shift occurs. When you truly love someone unconditionally, you love that person in a way he wants to be loved. Recognition of love in a way you are comfortable showing it is not a condition. The five love languages are:

- Words of Affirmation
- Acts of Service
- Quality Time
- Receiving Gifts
- Physical Touch

Anyone trying to strengthen a relationship with a child, spouse, parent, friend, or co-worker should take the time to find out that person's love language.

Amanda: Remember that people enjoy all of the five love languages, but we each have a primary love language that is the most important in relation to feeling understood. If your kids are too young to take the assessment online, you can usually tell what is most important to them by just watching to see what they do most often. This may change as they are figuring themselves out, so a helpful suggestion is to mirror what your child has done most recently.

Mike: This tool was an eye opener for me, because now I understand Amanda. I used to joke that in order to get some action, all I had to do was clean the house. Now it makes sense, because her strongest love language is acts of service!

It's quite amazing to see how far a small act like taking out the garbage without being asked goes toward strengthening the relationship and bond with your significant other. This one little piece of information has transformed my marriage for the better. It's really powerful for your kids, too. Stop and think about how simple this really is. I show my wife unconditional love, which means that I don't sweat the small stuff, in a way that resonates with her, by helping around the house or with the kids. These two simple changes have been life changing for our relationship. Today, I not only get more mommy/daddy time in the bedroom, she also encourages me to have fun with the guys on the golf course. This was not always the case.

At this point, you're probably asking yourself why we keep talking about love and respect in the same breath. The reason is because different people want different things. In addition to the five love languages, it is important to understand how love and respect complement each other. Many women will tell you the most important thing is love. But, let's be honest, many men want to be respected more than anything else. Remember the line from the Bronx Tale, when C asks Sonny, "Is it better to be loved or feared?" Sonny says, "It's nice to be both, but it's very difficult, but if I had my choice I would rather be feared." I'm not necessarily saying people would rather be feared than loved, but it does get the point across on how masculine energy is different from feminine energy. Ultimately, many people who identify with masculine energy feel love through being respected.

Amanda: I always feel like I have to jump in here and explain that we are not suggesting that women should become subservient to their husbands. That's not it at all. But the truth is that men and women are built differently, with different intrinsic energies. Typically, masculine energy is action-oriented and focused. Men are providers and protectors. Whereas feminine energy is intuitive, nurturing, visionary, and accepting. In fact, these energies complement each other, like yin and yang.

The interesting thing is that each person is a mix of both of these energies. Some men find themselves in more of a feminine energy role and some women take on more of a masculine energy role. There is no wrong or right, but when parents can each be aware of the other's energies, and work in harmony to balance each other, children feel understood, safe, protected, and nurtured. This method of balance works for a variety of family types, and there are ways for same sex couples to provide the complementary dynamic for their families the same as traditional families.

The great thing is that it only takes one person to put in motion a cycle of increasing love and respect, and then the two emotions fuel each other. When a man shows love to his wife, she receives his love and automatically shows more respect to her husband. Let's face it, what woman doesn't respect a man who is loving to his spouse? The great thing is that the spiral keeps building from there. If a woman shows respect to her husband first, he will respond by showing more love in return.

For example, when Missy showed respect to her husband, Mark, by commenting on what a great dad he is because he took the time to build a derby car with his son for cub scouts, he later showed her love by offering to give the kids a bath before bed. Her primary love language is acts of service, by the way!

Another example is how John showed love to his wife, Karen, by bringing home a really nice fur scarf after returning from a guys' getaway ski weekend. She instinctively returned the sentiment by expressing how thankful she was to have him home, because she felt safer when he was in bed next to her. She showed her respect for his role as protector of their family and both of them felt deeply connected.

It's very important to be mindful of the way we treat each other in a relationship because it only takes a simple act to start the spiral moving forwards. Then again, you have to watch out because it only takes a simple act to reverse the cycle as well. Sometimes even just a comment can throw the whole relationship into a backward spiral.

I'll never forget the day that I came home from running errands to see that Mike had cleaned the house. I felt thankful for his effort in cleaning our house, but, rather than showing respect right away for the work he did, I caught a glimpse of the stove top and said, "Thanks honey for trying, but how did you clean this?" It sounded totally disrespectful to him, and he responded with a very angry response, "Man, do you ever stop nagging?" I'll never forget it because this situation affected both of us for a day and a half. I was so mad, and didn't understand why Mike was so unloving, when I was only trying to help him see how to clean the stove better, and he couldn't believe how unappreciative of his efforts I had been.

One of the most transformative books for our relationship was *Love and Respect: The Love She Most Desires; The Respect He Desperately Needs*[8] by Emerson Eggerichs. I would suggest it to anyone who is looking to strengthen a marriage. As we mentioned in Step 1, having parents on the same page and showing love to each other has a huge impact on children's health and happiness.

Mike: One thing that I want to add here is that we talk about how important it is to show our family love and respect, because it helps to build a child's self-esteem. But what if you're not sure how your child is feeling about himself on the inside? Some parents say that their child seems happy, but ask how they can I gauge the child's overall health. Child therapist Alicia Birong shares how a child's behavior toward others is a good indication of what they feel about themselves. In other words, how your child acts is a reflection of what they see in themselves.

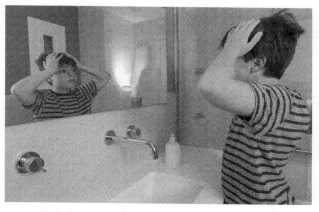

Your child's behavior can give you a glimpse of how much self-love they have. Alicia talks about three behaviors in particular to keep an eye on, because they may indicate low self-esteem. These behaviors are procrastination, high-risk decision-making, and excessive talking. This is important, because if a child doesn't have a lot of self-love, ultimately it will cause negative thoughts and feelings, which we will discuss in more detail later.

Another perspective to keep in mind is how we teach our children to show love and respect through personal responsibility. Therapist Lynn Barrett shares with us some helpful strategies for teaching your children how to take responsibility for their behavior. When a child shows disrespect to someone, it is helpful to pause, take a step back, and think what is a natural consequence for the behavior? Lynn told us about a time when her daughter was younger, when she kicked and spit at her. Instead of getting emotional and responding with anger, shock or frustration, she remained calm and simply told her daughter to go to her room. After a few minutes, she explained how, as a result of her actions, she wouldn't be able to join the family on a fun outing to the museum because a person who might kick or spit is not showing adequate responsibility to behave in a public place. Making difficult sacrifices, like rearranging anticipated plans, shows your children how important their behavior choices are. The hard part for parents is to remove our emotions. If we do, and are able to rationally allow our children to accept responsibility for their actions, and then show empathy for their feelings, we can teach valuable lessons in both love and respect.

When you take a moment to really understand yourself and the people in your family, you know what is important to feel loved, and it's pretty easy to be happier together. When parents remember **Change #3 – How We Learn**, showing acceptance and compassion to themselves, have the patience to learn what others' primary love language is, and then recognize how the balance of love and respect feed each other – it's common sense. When you approach LOVING and respecting your family unconditionally, you'll notice:

- Your child's self-esteem improving because they feel loved and understood for who they are

- Deeper connections with your spouse than ever before, as a result of your understanding of each other

- That you enjoy spending more time together as a family

Kelly: I can understand even more how to know my children better to help them feel loved. And, of course, that boosts their self-confidence.

Mike: It's really amazing how our kids learn to understand themselves better, too, and then they feel more in control. When a child feels empowered, everything changes.

Step 3 – LOVE and Respect Your Family – Bonus Resource Guide includes:

- Video with author Allen Vaysberg discussing tips for improving self-love

- Link to The 5 Love Languages Quiz

- Video of our daughters sharing their own love languages

- Video of child therapist Alicia Birong discussing signs of self-esteem in your child's behavior

- Video with therapist Lynn Barret discussing the importance of personal responsibility as a way to learn love and respect

Download here: www.hinmans/BonusRG.com.

Chapter 8

SLEEP Yourself to Health

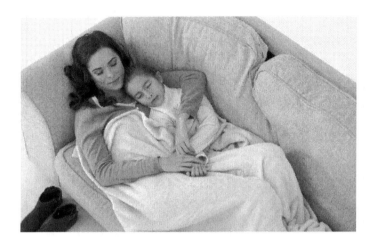

Kelly: This is really giving me so much to think about that I had never considered before. We've covered SEE how you prioritize health, FEED your body well, and LOVE and respect your family unconditionally. What's next?

Amanda: The next step is SLEEP yourself to health. What thoughts creep up when you hear about sleep for your child? You might think, "My child probably would feel better if he slept more, but he's never been a good sleeper." Or, maybe your first thought was, "My son crashes at night, because he's so active during the day, so this isn't an issue for us."

Sleep, or downtime, has become an underrated part of our fast-paced society. We all feel crunched for time; there is never enough time to fit in all the things we want to do. In our rush to DO, we have forgotten that one of the most important ways to support health and happiness, is to just BE. Said another way, we all need down time.

Mike: To be fair, you don't necessarily have to sleep to have down time, but plenty of deep sleep is always the best way for a body to heal and maintain optimal health. I can say that prioritizing my sleep was probably the biggest overall impact in healing from my anxiety. I used to wake up at 4:30 every morning for work, and would be up trading in the middle of the night on top of that. Lack of sleep was a huge part of my health challenges.

Amanda: To understand why this is so important, let's talk about the nervous system. We touched upon the two different modes of functioning of our nervous system earlier, when discussing cravings for sugar and self-love. The two modes are sympathetic and parasympathetic. The sympathetic nervous system is your fight or flight response (think adrenaline rush). When this system is activated, your body is busy releasing a flood of hormones, such as adrenaline, norepinephrine, and cortisol, into your blood. These hormones create a cascade of chemical reactions inside your body. For example, your blood vessels constrict to pump blood to the heart and large muscles (primarily in your hips and shoulders); your eyes dilate; and your sensory perceptions increase dramatically. All senses (vision, hearing, taste, smell, and touch) are on high alert; it's like someone cranked up the volume. We typically think of the five physical senses here, but it's important to note that a child's sixth sense is activated in a more amplified way, as well. A sixth sense is intuition, or a person's ability to energetically feel what emotions are in the environment around them. In general, kids have a very high level of perception of the sixth sense, even though they can't explain it. Think of it like this: Even if you never said a word about what you are feeling, your child has an ability to sense when you feel excited, joyful, calm, worried, overwhelmed, or anxious. It's like you have a neon sign over your head announcing all of your feelings to them.

Kelly: Wait a second, so you're saying my kids are aware of when I am feeling calm and when I'm feeling overwhelmed, even when I don't say anything about it?

Amanda: Yes. Not only are they aware of it, but chances are they are feeling it in a magnified way. Think about all the times when you are feeling some type of negative emotion like worry, being rushed, anxiety, frustration, and so on…they sense it too.

When the light switch is turned on, your child's body is in fight or flight response, and the volume is turned way up on all six senses. In other words, it's easier to see, hear, feel, taste, smell, and intuitively sense what's happening around you. Now, this is helpful when your child is playing in a basketball game, taking a test, or even playing Minecraft. It makes them more alert and sharp. The problem occurs when these chemical reactions are activated all the time!

The reason it is harmful to have your light switch turned on all the time is because it means that your body is not giving much attention to other important systems that are supported during parasympathetic nervous system activation, like your digestion, immune support, and reproductive system. In addition, this is when the emotional stability and creative centers in the brain are engaged as well.

Mike: When your child's light switch is turned off, his body is able to grow, rebuild, fight off infections and viruses, stay emotionally stable and think innovatively. When our kids were younger, we couldn't go a day without some major breakdown or temper tantrum. I just chalked it up to having girls. Now, we do still have those moments in our house, but they are significantly less frequent. Today, we know what to do to help our kids remember how to reorganize their nervous systems and calm down faster. And no, I'm not talking about NyQuil!

Kelly: This is really making me think about Kate. She is so reactive to situations, and I never understood why everything is such a big deal to her. I assumed this is the way she is, and always will be. Am I understanding correctly that when her light switch is turned on her body is more sensitive on purpose? And there is something we can do to help turn her light switch off, which will allow her to be less reactive?

Amanda: That's exactly right. It's common sense when you stop and think about it. Imagine you just left the spa after an hour long massage and pedicure with friends. Then you return home, and find your son pestering his sister to play catch with him. You are feeling relaxed and happy, so you may offer to play with him, instead.

Now switch the scenario, and imagine that you've finished a stressful day at work, where a project you've been working on for a month wasn't delivered to the client on time, your commute home was long because of an accident, and you return home to find your son pestering his sister to play catch with him. Chances are, you are not going to react the same way; in fact, you may even yell at him to leave his sister alone. The reason for these two completely different responses is because your body is literally different. The internal chemical balance is completely different. When a person is chronically on, it often leads to anxiety and has significant impact on interactions with others, most notably our loved ones.

To add to the importance of remembering to turn off your light, do you ever notice how many people today suffer from digestive distress; reproductive problems; and immune-related diseases, such as auto-immune conditions, cancer, and diabetes? What about the number of people struggling with emotional challenges? A large part of the reason is because most people live in sympathetic nervous system response (light switch turned on) almost all the time, and don't allow their bodies to support other systems.

Remember early on in the book when I said the number one question we hear is "How can I get my kids to eat better?" This is probably the single largest factor. The reason is because the sympathetic nervous system runs primarily on glucose, and the parasympathetic nervous system uses fat as the primary source of fuel.

Consider this perspective: What if there is nothing wrong with your child's craving for sugary food? In fact, what if his body were doing the BEST thing it could, considering the environment? If we dig a little deeper to uncover the Level 3 Why for a child's junk food cravings and lack of interest in eating more nourishing foods, it is often related to their nervous system. Sure, kids like the taste of some foods more than others, but there is a physiological reason your child's body is craving sugary and salty foods. It's because they provide quick sources of energy. When the light switch is turned on chronically, it requires a large amount of glucose, because the volume is turned up on all of your child's senses, which means the brain is processing a lot. The brain runs on glucose, so it only makes sense that they want sugar!

No matter how much we try to educate our kids about what is healthy for them and what is not, we will never trump their body chemistry. The only solution is to work with their bodies' natural processes by helping them learn how to turn their light switches off to support physical and emotional growth, immunity, and fat burning (parasympathetic mode).

Kelly: So, when my daughter's light switch is turned on, she is more sensitive to things around her, because the volume is turned up on all of her senses. That means her brain is working harder to process everything, so she is burning a lot of sugar. No wonder she wants to snack on cookies, goldfish, and fruit snacks all the time, but I can never get her to eat healthier foods. This could become a real problem, because it leads to anxiety. What kinds of things cause a person's light switch to be turned on?

Mike: Before I answer that, I want to point out that there is nothing wrong with having your child's light switch on. In fact, our bodies thrive in many situations when they are on. However, the problem is when we don't take the time to turn it off afterward. Balance is key.

Here are three common things that turn kids' lights on (sympathetic response):

- Activity – any type of physical activity or large movement

- Feeling strong emotions – experiencing things like joy, love, excitement, exhilaration, anxiety, being overwhelmed, fear, or despair

- Eating foods that contain sugar (including natural sweeteners) and stimulants, such as caffeine – this causes a flood of hormones in the body (anytime a person eats foods containing more than five grams of sugar per serving, according to Karen Hurd, RN)

Drs. Quintin and Katie Sleigh from Sleigh Family Chiropractic share with us how they see an increasing percentage of kids in their practice showing signs of excessive sympathetic nervous system response due to stress in school, busy schedules, and social influences. They remind us that stress is relative, so a child feeling worried about a test at school or being picked on at the playground can have the same impact as an adult's stress about paying the mortgage or finishing a project at work. They share how some of the changes in how we live are impacting our kids. For example, many kids have more hours of extracurricular activities, have more stimulation from devices, and less off time. Even bullying can follow kids home with social media and texting, which is different from a generation ago. All of these things demonstrate why it is so important to lead by example and teach your kids how to have down time.

Kelly: Now I know what to keep an eye on for both of my kids when their light has been on. What can I do to help them turn it off?

Mike: It sounds like you have a good understanding of the two sides of the nervous system. Here's how we can help our kids remember to turn off the light. Sleep is very beneficial for health, so making sleep a priority for your kids is important. A great strategy to help your kids sleep is to use a winding down process before bed. Find out what is relaxing for them. Maybe it's a massage, reading, talking, or cuddling. That's right, I said cuddling. I have four young daughters at home, so cuddling is a real thing in our house, and is used quite often. Try and avoid things that are stimulating, like screen time, bright lights, loud music, physical activity, and sugary foods.

Another easy tool you can use anywhere, anytime is breathing. Deepak Chopra teaches about the importance of breathing to calm the body and mind. When you stop to bring attention to your breathing, it changes; and when you take deep breaths, you automatically turn your switch off. Try taking eight Ujjayi breaths, or yoga breaths. This is where you inhale deeply through your nose and then with your mouth closed exhale through your nose while constricting your throat muscles. Tell your kids it sounds like Darth Vader from Star Wars.

Change 2 – How We Live

In addition to avoiding stimulation before bed, you can intentionally decrease a number of stimuli in their environment throughout the day. At the beginning of the book, we shared how the amount of information that a typical person processes in a 24-hour period today is the same as what our parents did in a year as kids. That means that our kids' brains are literally sorting through more information in one year than our grandparents did in their entire lives. Kind of gives you a new perspective on why so many children today struggle with maintaining attention.

Removing or decreasing the noises, smells, tastes, feelings, and sights in our kid's daily lives provides a chance for their brains to relax and makes it easier to switch the lights off. Some practical strategies include:

- Remove scented candles, plug-ins, or other strong-smelling items, especially in their bedrooms.

- Pay attention to noise in the environment and either turn down or turn off TVs, music, barking dogs, other siblings. Sometimes this means encouraging a child to take time away from the action and relax on their own.

- Avoid strong flavors in food, especially spicy foods. If your child prefers only bland foods, chances are it's related to an overtaxed nervous system. Many people find that when they're able to switch the lights off, their taste buds change drastically.

- Be mindful of fabrics, textures, seams, etc., in your child's clothes and shoes. This is especially important for things that have direct contact with skin for long periods of time.

- Monitor the amount of screen time from TVs, tablets, phones, etc. The more pixels, the more work for the brain. Limiting screen time before bed is statistically proven to improve sleep habits.

Kelly: You just gave me so much information and a new perspective. I'm interested in trying some of these things and seeing how they impact my daughter. When you mentioned a calming-down routine before bed, it reminded me of what I used to do when she was a baby. When my kids were little, we had a routine of bath and then reading before bed. I guess I didn't realize how much of that has kind of slipped away. We still read together sometimes, but not as often as we should, and I definitely never thought of reducing TV time or the cookies they always want before bed to help them sleep. The crazy thing is that my kids love TV and I always thought it seemed to calm them down. I wonder why that is.

Amanda: People often think, if my child is over-stimulated, why do they enjoy watching TV so much? Or why do they love the smell of the scented candles in our house? The reason is because the sensory processing in our brains acts like a pendulum. Our bodies are trying to balance when the volume is turned way up, and we reach overload, so the nervous system tries to regulate by turning everything down really low. Then the body registers minimal external sensations and starts to seek input. In other words, the pendulum swings back and forth from high to low, instead of maintaining balance in the middle.

A great way your child can regulate their nervous system and balance in the middle is by doing some type of large gross motor movement. When your kids are really worked up about something and feel very upset or angry, remember a huge burst of adrenaline is rushing through their blood. That hormone is released because their bodies are preparing to either fight or flee, so they are doing exactly what comes naturally by acting out in a demonstrative way. Instead of trying to squelch the energy or talk to them rationally, like I used to do, give them a pillow to hit, or do 15 jumping jacks with them.

When you show them that you understand what is happening in their body, that it's not something they can control in the moment, because the emotional stability part of the brain is not getting any attention, and then offer help, it is amazing how quickly things can turn around.

Kelly: I can already see how I will look at Kate's strong reactions in a different way. Instead of getting frustrated, and not understanding why she is so out of control, I can help her release her energy by doing jumping jacks or something with her. It feels good to have a deeper understanding of what is going on in her body and learn about things that may help her.

Amanda: It's really eye-opening for parents to learn and understand this. I love how Nick Ortner, CEO of The Tapping Solution, talks about our different modes of operation. He says our best resources, the rational, creative thinking and emotional stability centers of our brain, are off-line when our light switch is turned on. We literally do not have access to the best parts of our brains when we are stuck in sympathetic nervous response. Many adults describe this as "foggy brain".

Kelly, I can understand what you are feeling about your daughter, because we had the same thing in our house. For me, this understanding allowed me to release a lot of guilt. It's almost weird to say this, but when my girls would react in such a big way, I thought something was wrong with my parenting. Maybe I wasn't clear enough with setting limits, or maybe I gave in too much. I didn't know why they reacted so strongly, but I assumed that it wasn't normal. Now I know that it's exactly what their bodies are telling them to do. It just gives me a heads up that there are other things we can look at to find balance in their lives. It's simply about helping them learn to turn off the light more often.

Right now we are going through an interesting learning curve in our house. Our oldest daughter, Julia is really pressing for a phone. We have had many conversations with her about the responsibility it takes to have a phone (think of all those extra pixels her brain will be working to sort through each day!) and be able to maintain balance in life. She is aware of the extra stimulation it will cause, so we talk about how she has to show that she is self-aware of when her light switch has been on too much and then take steps to turn it off. For example, when she has a long day at school or didn't get a chance to eat nourishing foods her pattern has been to pick on her sisters by touching them or commenting on something she knows will frustrate them. She has been working very hard on recognizing when she feels agitated and instead of bugging someone else she will go jump on the trampoline, write in her journal, play piano or do tapping.

We also set a standard that phones get plugged in to charge in our kitchen, so they don't go upstairs to bed with us and she already knows that even after she eventually gets a phone it is not a permanent thing. Mike and I place a high priority on her health and explained that if we notice it having a negative impact on either her emotional of physical health the privilege will be removed until she is back in balance. Now to be fair, we talked about how we want the same health for ourselves, so if she notices that we become cranky, short-tempered or sees other negative side effect from having our light switch on too much, we ask that she bring it to our attention. We will see how this plays out, but both of us have been very clear about expressing our intentions for supporting health and happiness as a top priority for everyone.

With a new understanding of **Change 2 – How We Live** in today's society, you begin to recognize when your child's light switch is turned on and when it is turned off, and then make choices to balance the two in your family's life. You'll notice:

- Your child will experience less sensitivity and reactive behaviors.

- Over time, your child and everyone else in your family will have diminished cravings for sugar and salty foods.

- Everyone in the family will feel less anxiety and worry.

Kelly: If you're telling me I will be dealing with fewer temper tantrums and crying fits, I'm in! I never thought about how things like noises and smells in our environment can impact how agitated people feel, including me.

Mike: Step 4 – SLEEP Yourself to Health – Bonus Resource Guide includes:

- Video with Drs. Quintin and Katie Sleigh discussing the impact of the two sides of our nervous system

- Video with three strategies to increase downtime for your family

- Information on Emotional Freedom Technique, or Tapping

Download here: www.hinmans/BonusRG.com.

Chapter 9

MOVE for Fun

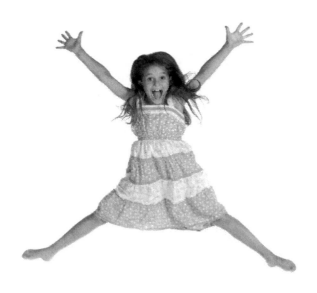

Kelly: This is really helpful information, and I love how you provide so many resources for me to learn more. I'm sure we are just hitting the surface of each of these topics, but already I feel like I understand my kids so much more. Is there more to consider?

Mike: Yes, we are off to a great start. We have three more steps to the Hinman Family Health

Method to share. Now that we just talked about how important it is to make time in your life to unwind and rest, it's time to talk about what type of activity is important for great health. Life is all about balance. You have to be living under a rock not to know that moving your body is an important part of living a healthy life. We are born with a desire to get going. Think back to your child when they learned to crawl, and then to walk. They are constantly moving!

Dr. Tommy John, from Tommy John Family Chiropractic, says, "Movement is like food for your brain." The reason is because when we move, our brains are using proprioception, (our body's own awareness in space) to process the environment. When your son jumps up and down, his inner ear, otherwise known as his vestibular system, kicks in so that he lands on his feet and absorbs the forces of gravity without collapsing. All of these different things are happening instinctively inside his body. He's not thinking about any of it, it just happens.

Amanda: When a person activates the instinctive processing in their brain, it draws energy or attention away from other things. Said another way, when your son is jumping up and down, he's not worried about being left out by his friends.

Also, movement can improve a child's ability to concentrate and focus. Kelly, you mentioned that your son loves to play sports, and I'd be willing to bet he's pretty good at them too.

Kelly: Yes, he is. Many times I've thought, too bad he doesn't love school as much as he loves baseball. It's amazing, because he can memorize all the stats of different baseball players and execute plays on the soccer field with ease, but when it comes to school he just doesn't seem to care. He hasn't had trouble with school, exactly, but he just wants to get it over with as soon as possible. Do you think it's because of the amount of activity?

Mike: There could be a lot of reasons why he would rather be playing baseball than learning science, but the amount of activity could definitely affect his ability to remember and stay focused. As we said before, physical movement helps regulate a child's nervous system. Studies show that when schools adopt regular movement breaks into the day, students' learning improves. In fact, Dr. Tommy John shares how even when people are aging and worried about Alzheimer's or another cognitive decline, sometimes they think of doing crossword puzzles or other mind sharpening puzzles, but studies prove that none of those methods are as effective as physical activity.

A strategy that helps some kids with homework time is to do a fun activity like jumping on a trampoline, running relay races, or riding a bike before sitting down to complete homework. It doesn't have to be long, just a few minutes makes a difference.

Kelly: Great idea! Homework time can be a battle with my son and I never thought about having him run around for a few minutes first.

Amanda: Movement will be helpful for your daughter too. Author Sharon Heller talks about the use of movement in her book *Too Loud, Too Bright, Too Fast, Too Tight; What to Do if You Are Sensory Defensive in an Overstimulating World*[9] as a tool to help balance people with a high level of sensory processing. This is how you can help your child balance, rather than have a pendulum swinging from high, to low, to high again. High-level sensory processing comes from having your light switch turned on most of the time. Many children have tremendous benefit from taking simple movement breaks similar to those in occupational therapy. Any kind of large movement works great, such as jumping jacks, climbing, crawling, handstands, etc.

Mike: On the other hand, while activity is great, anything in excess is not. It is possible for the amount or type of activity in a child's life to cause problems too. We learned this the hard way. Before our daughter developed seizures, she was involved in competitive gymnastics, competitive cheerleading, chorus, dance, and piano – all at age eight. Looking back, I think to myself – duh – no wonder her brain just needed to shut off! It was too much stimulation for her little body.

Our simple technique for determining if your child has a healthy balance of activity is to ask, "Is it fun?" Ask your child do you like hockey practice, swim lessons, dance team, etc. We are not saying go quit the team if they didn't enjoy a practice here and there, but in general, follow your child's lead to find out what they are interested in. Trust in the fact that when your child feels loved and supported for who she is, her body is getting all of the essential nutrients it needs to work well and make good parts, and she doesn't feel overwhelmed because her light switch is turned on all the time, she will naturally want to move and have fun in a healthy amount.

Amanda: There is a great opportunity to enjoy more fun time together as a family. Find activities that you all like to do. There are tons of different ways to be active. Perhaps you can try something new, like yoga stretches, or dance to your favorite song with your kids.

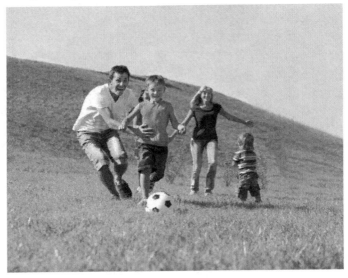

It doesn't have to be a big elaborate plan, sometimes the last minute walk to the park or soccer game in the backyard is the most fun. When you understand **Change #2 – How We Live**, you create plenty of space for movement in your family life, whether it be walking the dog, going for bike rides, etc. You give a gift of health to your kids and yourselves. Chances are your children will jump at the chance to move, especially if you are involved. When you keep fun as a focus for activity, you will enjoy:

- Stronger focus and mental clarity for your child and family.

- Feeling energized and vibrant – no more lethargy or exhaustion.

- Enjoying new experiences together as a family, including activities that you enjoy, rather than doing things you feel like you have to do.

Kelly: Your approach to exercise is different, and it makes sense. It's interesting because you don't even really talk about it as exercise, which can feel like a chore.

Mike: That's exactly right; we want to inspire families to include activity as part of their daily lives, but it doesn't have to be the regular 60-minute workout at the gym, or an organized sports class. Those things are fine and do provide benefits to your health when they are things you enjoy, but the reality is that if either one starts to feel like an obligation, it's probably causing more harm than good.

Change 2 – How We Live

We have been programmed to think you have to have a specific workout routine or keep your kids involved in organized sports for their health. If you look back over history, although sports have always been a part of society, the amount and type of activity has changed dramatically. Many kids today are involved in numerous activities, and practice countless hours. Of course, there are all sorts of benefits to being involved with sports, like socialization, teamwork, learning persistence, etc. But strictly talking about the benefits of the activity itself, it is actually more beneficial to take ten, five-minute movement breaks throughout your day than it is to sit all day and workout in one session. Your brain craves movement consistently. So just listen to your body, stand up, move, and stretch when it feels good!

Kelly: I'm going to keep that perspective. To be honest, it feels like you gave me permission to be a little easier on myself.

Amanda: Yes! This is key. We should be easier on ourselves, because - let's be honest – there are many adults who don't make activity a priority in their lives. When the belief about what type and how much activity is stuck into a box that doesn't fit into our lives, we don't do it. Wouldn't you rather show an example to your kids of how to stay active and have fun for the rest of your life? This is a really impactful message, especially for young girls and boys, who can become concerned about body image. When they see their parents being active in a healthy way, eating real foods, demonstrating their own self-love, and having a positive mindset, which we will talk more about in the last step, they learn by example and avoid body image challenges.

Kelly: It's interesting, because again I find myself thinking very differently about things. It's amazing how much there is to consider when I'm presented with new perspectives.

Mike: That is exactly what Amanda and I want to provide for parents – a chance to think about things differently and discover what is impacting their children's lives. Keep what you learn here in mind, and then see how it relates to your family. Don't take our word for it, see if it resonates with your situation.

Kelly: Sounds fair, I appreciate the fact that you always defer to me as a parent to know what is best for my family.

Step 5 – MOVE for Fun – Bonus Resource Guide includes

- Video with Dr. Tommy John discussing the impact of movement and brain function

- Kids yoga video with sample stretching, breathing, and movement exercises, which help regulate the nervous system.

Download here: www.hinmans/BonusRG.com.

Chapter 10

BELIEVE It Is Possible

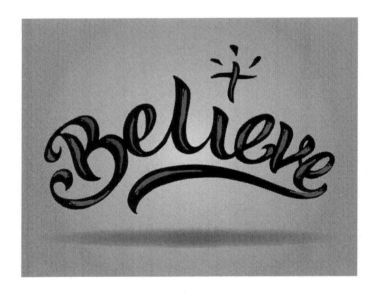

Kelly: There are two more steps in the Hinman Family Health Method. What's next?

Amanda: The next step is to BELIEVE it is possible. We will share why a person's beliefs are so meaningful. To start, I want to say that we seriously thought about putting this step at the start of the program; it's that important. But we realized in our own journey that deep faith is something that takes a while to develop, especially when you are in the middle of a tough situation with your child. It's hard to believe that there may be a reason for this circumstance, and that there is a great lesson that can be learned from it.

The first five steps of our method get you in touch with your body, and your child's body, on a deeper level than you have ever known before. When you learn the Level 3 Why things are the way they are, what you can do to find balance, and then begin to see changes happening, it is easier to believe that anything is possible. Believe that it is possible to heal from allergies, live free from anxiety, cure seizures and auto-immune conditions, feel loved for who you are, be connected on a deep level, anything.

In fact, Dr. Lissa Rankin talks about the importance of the power of your beliefs in her book, *Mind Over Medicine: Scientific Proof You Can Heal Yourself.*[10] She puts forth that a patient's belief in his ability to heal is the single most important factor in determining if they will in fact heal; second only to surrounding themselves with a support network that shares the same belief. Lissa Rankin is an MD who spent years practicing in traditional medicine and became curious about why some of her patients would receive care and information about their diagnosis and heal, while others received the same care and information, but didn't. She then dedicated her time studying case studies of spontaneous remissions and cures, and found a common link to people who healed. It was their belief in the possibility of recovery, as well as if they were surrounded by a supportive network, including caretakers, doctors, and loved ones who believed it too. We will talk a little more about the power of your thoughts and how they influence what happens in your life in Step 7.

Kelly: You're saying that Dr. Rankin examined case studies of people who healed from incurable diseases, and it was because of their faith?

Mike: I can hear the skepticism in your voice, and have to admit that this step was the hardest for me. In fact, I still struggle with it. Believing that everything happens for a reason and the Universe has your back, no matter what, is a pretty big concept to wrap your mind around. I'm a facts and stats kind of guy. I need to see the proof and don't believe something just because someone says "trust me".

I also read Dr. Lissa Rankin's book too and even though she shared evidence of case studies about spontaneous remissions, I still had a hard time believing that this was entirely because of the subjects' faith. Let's be honest, you can't see how much faith someone has, it's not easily measured or compared, and that means it's hard to prove. But for me to take the leap of faith, and believe in a higher power, really came down to one of two choices. I could work on growing my faith, and if it did have an impact, my chances of a successful outcome are higher. Or I could dismiss faith, and be left with learning to live with a situation I didn't want. In other words, even if I can't understand it or prove it exactly, I realize my life can only be better by taking a leap of faith.

Kelly: Mike, I'm with you. It's hard to trust something that you can't see or logically prove. But you make a good point when you say that by taking a leap of faith, it gives a sense of optimism, if nothing else, which is always a good thing.

Change 3 – How We Learn

Amanda: When we talk about faith, we are referring to some type of spiritual practice. There are many different ways that people incorporate spirituality into their lives. Some people have a deep sense of faith cultivated through a formal religion; others find a spiritual connection in nature or art; still others practice mindfulness through yoga and meditation. It is not our place to debate what type of spiritual practice is best for your family. That is up to you to decide. While the number of people who are religiously unaffiliated has increased to 22.8%, according to a 2014 PEW Research Religious Landscape poll, a majority of adults still report being spiritual in some regard. However, there is an interesting sentiment to reflect upon. It has been argued that by remaining spiritual, but not religious, people are less likely to openly discuss and practice faith in their daily lives. It is important to keep in mind that if parents have a spiritual faith themselves, but do not openly share, display, and teach their children about it, a lack may appear in their children's lives. Overwhelmingly, the verdict is that when people believe in a higher power, they find synchronicity and purpose in life, and as a result, their health and happiness are enhanced.

Don't get me wrong, I understand that this is tough to do, especially during hard times. During the dark months, when our daughter was having daily seizures, I could not comprehend how this situation could have a silver lining. All I focused on was keeping her safe and trying to figure out how to help her heal. It wasn't until we were through the hardest part that we realized the information we were uncovering about how to balance her body would not only help her, but dramatically improve our entire family's health and happiness. The amazing thing is that it has created a ripple effect, and now we are able to help thousands of other parents and children. My hope in sharing this with you is to inspire you that there is a silver lining to your situation too.

What's really amazing is the fact that most kids have an easier time believing in the possibility of incredible things than we do. Think of how they soak up all the joy and excitement that comes with their belief in Santa.

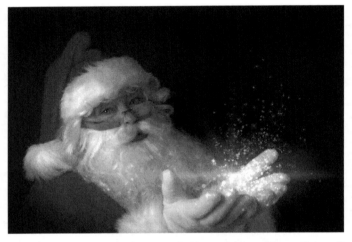

As parents, we understand the magic of how this all happens, but in reality it, doesn't matter to your children if they understand all of the logistics. They simply take the leap of faith and accept the fact that they don't know all of the answers to how Santa can deliver toys to everyone in one night. Because of their strong faith, the result is special. It's funny, because when we become adults we lose the humility to recognize that we don't have to know all the answers. It's like we are scared of being wrong.

Our daughters have provided many recent examples of the power of positive belief. We talk about how important belief is with our girls all the time, and celebrate moments when their strong belief paid off. Last fall, Julia became interested in learning how to make sushi. She asked if Mike or I knew how to do it, and if we could teach her. Neither one of us did, but we encouraged her to keep thinking about how she could come up with a way to learn. Two weeks later, we were grocery shopping at Marianno's and saw a sign posted for a sushi and sake night. Sure enough, Julia eagerly learned how to make a spicy tuna roll the next week, and Mike enjoyed the sake!

Another example happened while visiting friends in Atlanta on our spring break trip. We had the day open to tour the city, and when asked what they would like to do, Isabel said she wanted to see animals and art. Those two things seemed pretty far-fetched, considering we were planning on walking around Centennial Olympic Park. When we arrived at the park we were shocked to see that there was a Purina One Dog Competition taking place, with open seats in the stands. The girls loved watching dogs run and jump into the water and perform tricks. Then, after a quick lunch, the girls had a bathroom break in the basement of the building, and we discovered a new interactive art museum that had just opened. Of course, we had to go through it, and we took fun 3D pictures. It was really incredible, and we couldn't have come up with those things if we tried. These are just two of the many fun stories that happen due to their strong power of belief.

We love the movie *Inside Out*, because it gives such a great illustration of the power of your thoughts. In the movie, the audience has a glimpse inside the thoughts of Riley, the main character. It provides an incredible way to talk to your child about how a person's thoughts and emotions shape their beliefs, and then how those beliefs translate into daily life experiences.

Kelly: You're saying our beliefs are important because they impact our daily lives. Are you suggesting that I take a closer look at my beliefs to see if they are helpful to our family?

Amanda: Yes, exactly. Can you think of any beliefs you currently have that you would like to adjust?

Kelly: I would like to believe that Kate isn't over-reactive, I want to believe that my kids are not picky eaters, and that Dylan is engaged and loves learning in school.

Mike: That's a great start! Here's a little exercise we use in our program to start a perspective shift. It's an exercise called "Because anything is possible, I want _____ in my life." There are many ways to use this exercise with your family. You can write it down and post it around your kitchen, take turns talking about it over dinner or breakfast. Whatever works for your family, just remember the more you reinforce positive belief, the more likely it is to become a reality!

Amanda: When you are able to keep in mind **Change 3 – How We Learn**, cultivate a deep sense of faith, and BELIEVE that all things are possible – and then empower your kids to believe too – you experience:

- Your child – and yourself – feeling hopeful that they can change difficult circumstances in life.

- Understanding that a part of life includes struggle, but now you accept the struggles, and even have a sense of gratitude for them, because you know there is an amazing potential for growth each time.

- Everyone in the family feeling more secure, loving, trusting, and optimistic.

Kelly: It's crazy to think that I can actually get to a place where I am thankful for the challenges in my life because I know there will be something I can learn from them.

Amanda: Yes, it may sound like this is too good to be true, but it is possible to get to a place where you can approach everything with a sense of gratitude and teach your kids how to look at life through that lens.

Step 6 – BELIEVE it is Possible – Bonus Resource Guide includes:

- "Belief is #1 Importance" video sharing discussion about Dr. Lissa Rankin's discovery of the power of our beliefs

- "Children's Belief" video shares real life stories of cultivating a positive belief and experiencing unexpected outcomes

- Because Anything is Possible PDF

Download here: www.hinmans/BonusRG.com

Chapter 11

CLEANSE Your Family's Stress

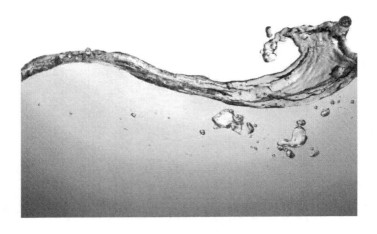

Kelly: We've covered everything from food, to love, to sleep, to activity, and to beliefs. I'm curious: What else is there?

Mike: This brings us to the last step in our Hinman Family Health Method, which is to CLEANSE your family's stress. Sounds kind of strange to cleanse your stress, right? Most people think of trying to reduce your stress or eliminate your stress. Well, the reason we say cleanse your stress is that you really just want to experience the good stress in your life, without too much of the bad stress. Stop and think about it; everything causes stress on our bodies. I mean, stress is simply pressure on an object. This is both positive and negative, but we tend to think of it as always negative. A hug is stress on the body, the excitement your child feels before her birthday is stress, laughing so hard that your stomach aches is stress! Obviously, we want to keep this type of stress.

Amanda: This is why we want to cleanse your family's stress, rather than get rid of it. In order to shift stress from negative to positive, we need to know where all the negative stress is coming from. I'm going to take you through four steps to understand the source of negative stress. Stick with me here, because it may be new for you, but it's so worth it once you grasp the potential to change your life!

Mike: I'm going to give you a little reader warning here. We are going to share a LOT of information in this section, and most of it may be new or even seem far-fetched, especially if it is the first time you are hearing it. It was for me. Please understand that it is our intention to provide you with some new perspectives to consider. Amanda and I are not here to convince you of anything, or lecture you on what to think. In fact, we would prefer it if you look into this topic and come to your own conclusions. That is why we feel strongly about providing you with many resources that were very valuable to us.

Kelly: Now I'm interested. How do our kids have negative stress?

Amanda: Ok, so let's talk about four steps to understanding where our negative stress comes from. This process is the same for adults and children. We are happy to share much of the information we learned from our mentor Fabienne Fredrickson at her amazing Mindset Retreat.

1. First, our brains create thoughts, and thoughts equal energy. Let's go back to the previous step, BELIEVE it is possible. Remember how Dr. Lissa Rankin dedicated years of her life to learning why some people healed from incurable situations and others didn't? She concluded that it was because of their beliefs about recovery, and here is why. Modern technology and the field of metaphysics help us understand that each and every thought is energy.

Brain mapping shows where and when different areas of a person's brain light up, and this is where energy is present. Another technology to witness the presence of energy in our brain is an EEG test. When our daughter was having seizures, doctors recommended this test, and they could literally see the amount and location of the energy in her brain.

2. The second key concept is energy attracts like energy. The Universal Law of Attraction states that our thoughts, feelings, words, and actions produce energies which, in turn, attract similar energies. Negative energies attract negative energies and positive energies attract positive energies. This is a Universal Law, which means it is always true. It is precisely why taking that leap of faith to have belief in the possibility of healing is so impactful. Because it literally attracts healing energy into your life.

3. Next, it is important to understand the difference between conscious and

subconscious thoughts. Susan Shumsky's quote is helpful to understand this distinction. She says, "Your conscious beliefs are what you THINK you believe. Your subconscious beliefs and deepest convictions are what you REALLY believe."

This is where it starts to get a little tricky, because people are aware of their conscious thoughts, but most people are unaware of their subconscious thoughts. However, your subconscious beliefs always create a larger percentage of the thoughts in your mind. In other words, your subconscious beliefs always win the inner struggle, because there is more energy coming from your subconscious thoughts than from your conscious thoughts.

4. Therefore, Step 4 is to align your subconscious thoughts with what you consciously want in life. This is called deliberate creation, and it's where amazing things happen! By deliberately creating positive beliefs in your subconscious mind, you will be attracting positive things into your life. That means we need to learn how to intentionally shape our subconscious beliefs.

Here's the amazing part - our subconscious mind MUST accept any image or thought that is presented. It cannot differentiate between what is real and what is imagined. This is very powerful, because the subconscious mind is NOT able to distinguish fact from fiction. Our subconscious minds are shaped by our actual *experiences* and *imaginations*.

Kelly: Let's see if I follow. Our thoughts and beliefs attract things into our lives. When I'm thinking positive things, then I will experience positive things, but when I'm thinking negative things, I will experience negative things.

Amanda: You got it!

Kelly: But what's a little tricky is that even if I say to myself, "Think positive thoughts", but my subconscious thoughts are still doubtful, I'm not really attracting positive things. Is that right?

Amanda: Yes, that's right, our subconscious thoughts are the ones we may not be aware of, but they are the most important.

Here's a story that helps illustrate the difference between our conscious thoughts and our subconscious thoughts. Whenever I asked my daughter Avery to clean her room, she would pick up the clothes and toys on the floor and tossed across her bed, and shove everything into her closet. Our conscious thoughts are like the things you see when you step into the room. Avery's room often appeared clean at first glance, but when I opened her closet, here's what I saw.

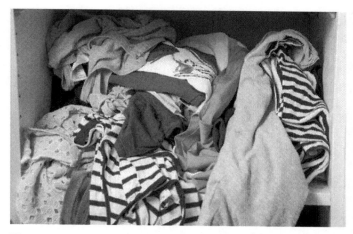

The reality is that if everything is shoved into the closet in a crumpled mess, it doesn't make her life easier to find her school uniform in the morning, or see where her leotard is for gymnastics. So when we talk about having a clean room, I ask, "Is it completely clean?", and she knows I'm referring to the inside of her closet, too. The same goes for our subconscious mind. If we only work on being aware of our conscious thoughts, we are ignoring all the stuff in the closet, and that is what really makes our life easier.

Kelly: You said that we can intentionally create subconscious beliefs using imagination, because information isn't limited to current facts, is that correct?

Amanda: Exactly! Our subconscious beliefs are formed by both actual *experiences* and *imagination*. So let's take a look at how we can attract positive beliefs through our experiences first. Remember in Step 2, LOVE and respect your family unconditionally, we shared the importance of learning to love yourself first? Most people focus more on the negatives than the positives when it comes to themselves. For example, when Trish snapped at her daughter to put her shoes on right now! I empathized with her situation, because I've been there and know how frustrating it can be to battle a fiercely independent two-year old, but when I do the same thing, I become self-critical of my parenting. This is why it's so important to love yourself first as an example to your children. Be compassionate and kind in your own self-talk, so your actual experiences are positively shaping your subconscious mind.

Change 3 – How We Learn

The other piece affecting the subconscious mind is imagination. Kids have a natural tendency towards creative play, which is very powerful. Anytime they imagine positive things, they are shaping their subconscious minds, which will ultimately attract positive things into their lives. Unfortunately, as kids grow up, structured time often increases, leaving less time for imagination and creativity. As we said at the beginning of the book, the average child today spends over 500 additional hours each year in structured activities than in the 1980s. The public education environment has changed dramatically in the past couple of decades. There is more structured time and less free exploration or creative learning, because of the focus placed on standardized metrics in education. Sir Ken Robinson gave the most popular TED talk ever, entitled "Do Schools Kill Creativity?", and it has reached over 38 million views on this subject. His argument is that we should be intentional about providing more real life learning experiences for our children.

Mike: The takeaway from all of this is: In order to bring more positive things into your life, your top priorities need to be feeling good about yourself and making time for creative exploration in your life.

In order for us to teach our kids how to create what they want for the future, we must show them how to be happy and creative. The best way to do this is to lead by example. It is easier for parents to accept that their young kids can spend time being happy and cultivating imagination, but many adults think they as adults don't have time for fun or creativity, because they have to earn a living. Allen Vaysberg, the author previously mentioned, shares how important it is to add something you love to your day, even if it's only ten minutes of painting, looking at pictures, walking outside or writing.

Just think, if you can find a way to add creativity and gratitude into each day, you are changing your subconscious beliefs, which CLEANSES your stress. The bottom line is this: your emotions are directly tied to your future.

Kelly: What you're saying is that when I allow my kids more unstructured time in their lives it is beneficial to their health?

Amanda: Absolutely. Unstructured, imaginative play is so valuable for our kids. I'm not just talking about young kids – this is important when they get older, too. Usually, the type of creativity shifts from imaginative play to something else, like journaling, building with Legos, painting or other art, making forts, filming movies, you name it. When our kids are passionate about things, they are tapping into their creativity. When they feel passionate and happy, they're attracting positive things into their lives.

However, be mindful that the reverse is true too. When kids' days are loaded up with structured time in school, extra-curricular activities and sports practices, where most of the decisions and expectations are dictated by someone else, they may be losing out on the positive development of their subconscious minds. Frequently structured activities are light switch on activities because they require focus, recall, physical movement or concentration to meet a predetermined goal where unstructured activities are light switch off activities because they tend to be more fluid, innovative and not defined.

In fact, a study from the University of Colorado Boulder found that "children who spend more time in less structured activities – from playing outside to reading books to visiting the zoo – are better able to set their own goals and take actions to meet those goals without prodding from adults." Yuko Munakata, a Colorado University-Boulder psychology and neuroscience professor, goes on to share that a study published online in the journal *Frontiers in Psychology,* also found that children who participate in more structured activities – including soccer practice, piano lessons, and homework – had poorer "self-directed executive function".[11]

Kelly: Sometimes my kids do love to just be left on their own and play creatively. But I have to be honest; other times that seems to be more stressful, because they don't know what to do, and end up picking on each other. What if the unstructured time causes more problems?

Amanda: I know what you mean. Sometimes it seems like more of a hassle to just leave our girls to their own devices. It does take a little practice for kids to know how to entertain themselves. Just like it takes some practice before Julia could learn how to do flip-flops, creativity is a skill that can be practiced. We have found it helpful to set some loose guidelines, explain that we expect respectful treatment of each other, set a time frame, and then let them see what comes up.

For example, when Mike and I wanted to spend a few hours working, and the girls had a day off school, we made time for creative play, with some basic guidelines. We explained that mom and dad would be busy working for two and a half hours, which means that we are available only for emergencies. The girls had access to the backyard for the first hour and a half, and then the basement for the last hour. They could take anything outside with them that they wanted to, and we would have lunch after, so no snacks until we were done working. Obviously, this was minimal structure, but it did give some boundaries around time, location, and food. The girls loved it and ended up making their own trampoline routine and a movie for us to watch later. You'd be surprised how much kids can amaze you when you provide an opportunity and belief that it will go smoothly.

Kelly: I'd like to try something like that with my kids. It probably helps to start out with a shorter time first.

Amanda: Yes, it's a good idea to practice and then increase unstructured time slowly. To recap, in order to shift the balance of stress your family feels to a positive rather than a negative, it is important to work on reshaping subconscious beliefs because it is these beliefs that are responsible for attracting everything in your life. Therefore, positive self-talk and making time for unstructured creativity in your child's life is effective. But the most important thing any parent can do is to lead by example. After all, our kids just want to be like mom and dad, at least until age ten or so!

The following is additional information to consider in relation to **Change 3 – How We Learn**. Remember how we talked in the beginning of the book about all of the specialists that are available now to help our kids, like pediatric endocrinologists, doctors that specialize in neurofeedback, occupational therapists, psychotherapists, and so on? The list goes on and on.

Our society is driven by the economy, which has become incredibly specialized. I saw this directly when touring various Illinois farms. One hundred years ago, farmers would grow a variety of crops and raise cattle, hogs, and chickens. Think of all of the depictions of farms in children's stories. But that is not the farming economy of the 21st century. Each farm specializes in one, or maybe two, things. It has become a very technical business. For example, corn farmers plot their land in grids and soil test every square meter of their land to determine the optimal type of seed, minerals, and fertilizer in order to maximize crop yield. However, by focusing on such a limited crop or specialized animal production, farms have lost the natural synergy that takes place when people, animals, and crops are in balance. These imbalances are responsible for many challenges in the industry that are beyond the scope of this book. But the message remains; too much specialization is detrimental, not only to business, but to our personal health, as well.

Another example is found in the medical profession. By the very nature of intense study, doctors are trained in specialized studies of medicine, and as a result, see things through the lens of familiarity. When Jack's mom took him to an ear, nose, and throat (ENT) doctor to see about his perpetual stuffy nose, ear infections, and snoring, he was told the best solution for his problems was to have his tonsils and adenoids removed. This seems logical for a specialist who is familiar with chronic infections, or even enlargement, of these glands. It is a procedure they perform frequently. However, by focusing on those areas of the body in isolation, there is a larger message that is being overlooked. The tonsils and adenoids are part of the body's immune system, and often are the first line of defense. As bacteria and viruses enter the body, they are responsible for alerting the immune system that an invader is present, so the immune system can mount a response and fight it off. If these glands are chronically infected or enlarged, it is a signal that the immune system is under constant pressure and is not functioning at optimal capacity. The Level 3 reason why a child may have chronic sinus infections, ear aches, and sore throats is because their immune system is not working well. You may recall back in Step 4, SLEEP Yourself to Health, we talked about the importance of turning your light switch off. If a child always has their light switch turned on, their immune system is not given much priority, so it is not able to function well. By ignoring the underlying cause, if no changes to Jack's lifestyle are made, then his body will continue to create new signals as a way of notifying him that his immune system isn't getting enough support.

These are just two examples of how failure to prioritize creative, imaginative time in our lives can have much larger ramifications. Practicing creativity helps us "think outside the box".

Kelly: You're saying that the farmer and the ENT doctor in your examples were not being creative, and that is what eventually leads to problems? I'm not sure I follow.

Amanda: Everything in life is about balance. We hear it all the time. That's why the analogy of a light switch is so helpful. An easy way to remember it is this: when a person's light switch is turned on, all six senses are turned up, and this has a focusing effect. So in cases when we want to be specific or detail oriented, it is very helpful. When a person's light switch is turned off, there is an opening, and energy is allocated to the creative, imaginative side of the brain. This is where innovation comes from. When a person, a company, an industry, or a society becomes imbalanced, problems arise. In life, we want to enjoy both precision and innovation, and by intentionally creating a balance, a child finds optimal health and happiness.

Kelly: This goes back to what I was learning before, about the light switch being turned on and off. Let's see if I understand what you're saying. When I am thoughtful about having down time for

Kate and Dylan, it's possible for their light switches to turn off. When their light is balanced, they will not only be healthier, but it also opens up their minds to imagination?

Amanda: Yes, I'm impressed! You have a great sense of how it all ties together. Can you see how this will help the original concerns you expressed about Kate being too sensitive and Dylan not that interested in learning?

Kelly: It's amazing because I can see how these things will help Kate be less reactive, and help Dylan be more open and creative in his learning.

Amanda: It's really powerful stuff! When your child loves himself, it is possible to cleanse his stress, which makes it easy to turn the light switch off on their nervous system, and reduce cravings for sugary, salty foods. Without the cravings, it's easier to choose nourishing food. By eating real foods, his body can build high-quality parts and feel naturally inclined to move for fun. When your child feels happy and healthy, it's easy to believe anything is possible!

Mike: I understand that this stuff may seem out of reach right now, but we wanted to put it all out there for you to consider. The possibilities on the other side are truly amazing! The great thing is that the amount of factual evidence to support what we just talked about continues to build as we understand more and more about the human brain, metaphysics, and universal laws.

But we don't want you to take our word for it. This is not the kind of thing you can just buy into because someone says it. We encourage our readers to look into this for themselves. Check out information from

John Assarf the founder and CEO of My Neurogym. He provides resources and programs that help a person transform his life from the inside out. He has termed this an "Innercise Revolution," and he understands life is short. You have big goals and dreams, and the years are passing. Imagine your life free of the things that are keeping you stuck and holding you back. We believe in the importance of this because as parents we are impacting our children every day as we lead by example. When parents are more optimistic and healthy, their children will follow.

Amanda: Yes, he has some great information. Another resource I would encourage our readers to look into is an incredible Mindset Retreat hosted by Fabienne Fredrickson. She has been very influential in our own personal growth and development. So I highly recommend it!

To quote U.S. Anderson, "When we finally realize that thought causes all, we will know that there are never any limits that we ourselves do not impose."

Mike: Amanda mentioned that this is not something you do once or twice, and then expect all of your life's challenges to disappear. Now that you are aware of **Change 3 – How We Learn**, it is possible to reshape your subconscious beliefs. It does take intention to add more creativity into your lives, but the possibilities are so great. Just to know that you can be in charge of what you create in your future is amazing. As a result of working on CLEANSING your family's stress, you will see:

- Your child grow up with a sense of gratitude.

- Your child learn appreciation for their own talents and abilities to take control of their future.

- Everyone in the family living with less anxiety.

Step 7 – CLEANSE Your Family's Stress – Bonus Resource Guide includes:

- Video with Allen Vaysberg discussing practical ways to increase love and creativity in your daily life

- Link to TED Talk with Sir Ken Richardson, in which he discusses the importance of unstructured, creative time as a way to develop and cultivate innovation

- Article and audio clip with Yuko Munakata where she discusses structured time vs. unstructured time, and the impact each has on development

- Information about My Neurogym created by John Assarf, where he shares many valuable resources and programs that help a person transform their life from the inside out

- Link to Fabienne Fredrickson's Mindset Retreat, where she teaches us how our thoughts, words, beliefs, and actions impact every aspect of our lives

Download here: www.hinmans/BonusRG.com.

Chapter 12

Putting It All Together

Kelly: You've taken me on a journey to see all of the things that can help my children's health. It's amazing to look back and see that we started by focusing on what the health priorities are for my family; then I learned so much about how food, love, sleep, and activity affect my kids. You even took it a step further to talk about how thoughts and feelings shape our lives. No wonder you were able to see such a transformation in your whole family.

After learning all of this information I have an idea of why three societal changes – **how we eat, how we live,** and **how we learn** – have an impact on our kid's health and happiness. I am putting together pieces of the puzzle, and I understand why Kate is sensitive and Dylan doesn't love learning in school. I also have an idea of what may be helpful for them and how we can start to include these things in their lives.

Amanda: There is so much that parents can learn about and take action on to help their children. The Hinman Family Health Method is a comprehensive system, and it provides amazing results. Do you remember the claim we made in the beginning: What if your child's diagnosis doesn't matter? Can you see how applying this same approach to a child with food allergies or a child with ADD can help them heal?

Kelly: It's crazy, because I can. My guess is both of these children probably have their light switch turned on too much, and if they were able to make changes, their bodies would function differently.

Amanda: That's exactly right! Please consider this information like a buffet, take what is helpful for you and move at your own pace. Every family is unique, and as Mom and Dad, only you know what is best for your kids.

Thinking back to when we were faced with challenges in our family, I felt so completely helpless, because it felt like there was nothing I could do to help my daughter. However, then I realized that there is so much that Mike and I could work on together with our daughter and for ourselves to become living role models for all of our children. That is why we created the Hinman Holistic Health Institute. We have dedicated our lives to sharing our message and providing support to other parents through a variety of platforms. We offer the Hinman Family Health Method™ coaching program for parents who are looking to enhance their children's confidence, concentration, and self-acceptance, as they improve their physical and emotional health. We also offer a Family Health Made Easy workshop which is a quick-start program that helps parents cut through the piles of information and focus on the most vital aspects of family health.

Kelly: I don't want this to be another book I read, and then don't do anything with the information. You know how sometimes you read a great book, even highlight things that you think will be helpful for you, but then instead of putting into practice, you put the book on some shelf somewhere and never apply all of the good advice you've gotten? I don't want that to be me, my family could really use support in implementing changes, especially because this is so new to me. How do you help parents who are interested in investing in their family's health and happiness now? Where can I learn more about your programs?

Mike: Thank you for bringing up an important question. Let's face it, not many of us can learn something one time and then seamlessly incorporate it into our lives. If you're like me, it's not that easy. If our message resonates with you, I encourage you to schedule a call today to talk about your own family's challenges, ask key questions, and talk about solutions, free of charge.

Go to **www.Hinmans.com/call** to schedule a free Health and Happiness Call today. Both Amanda and I would be happy to connect with your family to see if one of our programs is a good fit.

We offer a variety of programs, because we understand that families have unique situations and are in different places. For most parents, the support they find in being part of a community of other parents who are working toward increasing their children's health and happiness is irreplaceable. Think back to when you had Dylan. How valuable was it to talk with other new moms about nap schedules and first foods?

Kelly: You're right, I had a great group of friends that I met after having him, and it was amazing.

Amanda: Many people work well in group situations, and it feels good to know there are other parents experiencing the same things you are. This support is very motivating, especially when families are making changes.

Another important element offered in our programs is accountability. When parents are serious about wanting to experience a shift in their family's life, having accountability makes a huge difference in the actual implementation of change. It's just like having a personal trainer at the gym. It may be out of your comfort zone to ask for help, but just like the workout that doesn't happen without the trainer, we often don't take steps that we want to without accountability. Our programs put all of this together, as well as take the time to go through the steps of our Hinman Family Health Method in more detail and help you create an amazing future for your family. As the saying goes, "A rising tide lifts all boats!" When you join our community, your family will be lifted to new heights.

I suggest you schedule a call today if support, community, and accountability would be helpful for you. Feel free to visit our website at **www.Hinmans.com** to find out more information about our services.

Here's a recap of the steps in the Hinman Family Health Method:

The Hinman Family Health Method

Taking a closer look at how we eat, how we live, and how we learn

1. SEE How You Prioritize Health

    a. Find out where your family is today – this includes consistency and overall priority of healthy habits.

    b. Recognize how parents are different and take time to understand yourself, as well as your spouse, so that you may work together effectively.

    c. Create a specific vision for your family in the future – what does a vibrant family life look like for you in one year, five years, ten years?

2. FEED Your Family Well

    a. Understand that the food supply has changed drastically – the priority is to eat real food.

    b. Our bodies need certain foods to make great parts – these include proteins, fiber, vitamins, minerals, and essential fats.

    c. Emphasize crowding out highly processed, "chemicalized", food-like substances, and replacing with real foods – educate your kids on how it benefits them.

3. LOVE and Respect Your Family Unconditionally

   a. Love yourself first – you have to fill your own cup before you can give to others – do this by practicing more compassion and patience with yourself.

   b. Learn how each person in your family feels love – consider five love languages; acts of service, physical touch, receiving gifts, quality time, and words of affirmation.

   c. Understand that men and women, boys and girls have different energies – show love and respect to your family.

4. SLEEP Yourself to Health

   a. Two different modes for our nervous system – light switch on or off – the key is to find balance.

   b. Having too many stimuli in our environment turns on the light switch, which causes increased cravings for sugar, caffeine, alcohol, etc.

   c. There are many ways to regulate your nervous system – sleep, decreased environmental stimuli, movement, breathing, tapping, etc.

5. MOVE for Fun

  a. Movement is food for your brain – our bodies crave movement, and it regulates our nervous system - so move often.

  b. Activity is supposed to be fun, rather than obligatory – keep in mind that our bodies want to move. If we enjoy it, it's a good fit for us; if we don't, it's time to reassess what will work better.

  c. When movement is fun, it becomes a natural part of your daily life and results in a life that promotes health and happiness.

6. BELIEVE it is Possible

  a. Belief in something is the number one most important thing – so be mindful of what your thoughts, words, and actions are, because they create your beliefs.

  b. Share your spiritual practice with your children – whether it be through formal religion, meditation, connection to nature, art, or yoga – the key is to share it rather than keep it internal.

  c. Take a cue from our kids, and cultivate a deep sense of belief – practice daily with a mantra, prompt, prayer, or other activity of your choice.

7. CLEANSE Your Family's Stress

    a. Recognize that your thoughts, words, feelings, and actions are energy, and attract like energy.

    b. Our subconscious minds are shaped by both actual experiences and imagination – therefore, creativity is an essential part of building a positive subconscious mind.

    c. Provide plenty of time in your child's daily life for creativity and lead by example as you include it in yours, as well.

References

1) Brogan, Kelly. *Mind of Your Own.* Place of Publication Not Identified: Harper Thorsons, 2016. Print.

2) Dr. Joseph Mercola. "Why Your DNA Isn't Your Destiny". n.p. *Mercola.com,* January 23, 2010.

3) Shetreat-Klein, Maya, and Rachel Holtzman. *The Dirt Cure: Growing Healthy Kids with Food Straight from Soil.* N.p.:n.p., n.d. Print.

4) Cover, Stephen R. *The 7 Habits of Highly Effective People.* London: Simon & Schuster, 2005. Print.

5) Johns Hopkins Medicine. "The Brain-Gut Connection". n.p. Hopkinsmedicine.com, n.d.

6) Vaysberg, Allen. *The New Love Triangle: Your Practical Guide to a Love Filled Life!* Place of Publication Not Identified: Human Potential Press, 2016. Print.

7) Chapman, Gary. *Five Love Languages.* S.I.: Jaico House, 2008. Print.

8) Eggerichs, Emerson. *Love and Respect: The Love She Most Desires, the Respect He Desperately Needs.* Detroit; Christian Large Print, 2010. Print.

9) Heller, Sharon. *Too Loud, Too Bright, Too Fast, Too Tight; What to Do if You Are Sensory Defensive in an Overstimulating World.* New York; HarperCollins, 2002. Print.

10) Rankin, Lissa. *Mind Over Medicine: Scientific Proof You Can Heal Yourself.* N.p.:n.p., n.d. Print.
11) Jane Barker. "Kids whose time is less structured are better able to meet their own goals, says CU – Boulder study". *University of Colorado Boulder New Center*, June 18, 2014.

About the Authors

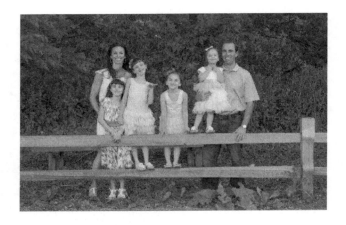

Mike and Amanda Hinman are the founders of Hinman Holistic Health Institute, Ltd. They work with parents who seek to maximize the health and happiness of their families. When their own family faced numerous health challenges they were blessed to come through the other side stronger than ever. That is why they have dedicated their lives to sharing what they learned about how to create a vibrant life for families. Their services include coaching, educational programs, seminars, speaking events and books as a way to support parents. They live in the Chicagoland area with their four young daughters.

33957108R00084

Made in the USA
San Bernardino, CA
15 May 2016